Meta-analysis in Medical Research

The handbook for the understanding and practice of meta-analysis

To those who have helped me become
who I am, even if they expected more

I am very grateful to Alberto Pilotto and Angelo Andriulli for many stimulating and thoughtful discussions on a number of theoretical and practical aspects of meta-analysis.

I am indebted to Giorgio Gasparro, DP man, for his patience with my requests.

A heart-felt thanks to Andrew K Burroughs, beacon of knowledge and wisdom for many people. Without his advice and support, this work would have never been written.

Meta-analysis in Medical Research

The handbook for the understanding and practice of meta-analysis

Gioacchino Leandro
Gastroenterologist, Biostatistician
Castellana Grotte, Italy

FOREWORD BY
Giuseppe Gallus
Head of the Institute of Medical Statistics
University of Milan, Italy

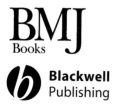

© 2005 Gioacchino Leandro
Published by Blackwell Publishing Ltd.
BMJ Books is an imprint of the BMJ Publishing Group Limited, used under licence

Blackwell Publishing, Inc., 350 Main Street, Malden, Massachusetts 02148-5020, USA
Blackwell Publishing Ltd, 9600 Garsington Road, Oxford OX4 2DQ, UK
Blackwell Publishing Asia Pty Ltd, 550 Swanston Street, Carlton, Victoria 3053, Australia

The right of the Author to be identified as the Author of this Work has been asserted in accordance with the Copyright, Designs and Patents Act 1988.

All rights reserved. No part of this publication may be reproduced, stored in a retrieval system, or transmitted, in any form or by any means, electronic, mechanical, photocopying, recording or otherwise, except as permitted by the UK Copyright, Designs and Patents Act 1988, without the prior permission of the publisher.

First published 2005

Library of Congress Cataloging-in-Publication Data

Leandro, Gioacchino.
  Meta-analysis in medical research : the handbook for the understanding and practice of meta-analysis / Gioacchino Leandro.
     p. ; cm
  Includes bibliographical references and index.
  ISBN 1-4051-2733-3 (alk. paper)
  1. Meta-analysis. 2. Medicine–Research–Evaluation.
  [DNLM: 1. Biomedical Research–methods. 2. Meta-analysis. 3. Bias (Epidemiology)
4. Publication Bias. WA 950 L437m 2004] I. Title.
  R853.M48L43 2004
  610′.72–dc22
                                                                            2004017776

ISBN 1-4051-2733-3

A catalogue record for this title is available from the British Library

Set in 10/13.5 Sabon by TechBooks, India
Printed and bound in India by Replika Press Pvt. Ltd.

Commissioning Editor: Alison Brown
Editorial Assistant: Claire Bonnett
Development Editor: Fiona Pattison
Production Controller: Kate Charman

For further information on Blackwell Publishing, visit our website:
http://www.blackwellpublishing.com

The publisher's policy is to use permanent paper from mills that operate a sustainable forestry policy, and which has been manufactured from pulp processed using acid-free and elementary chlorine-free practices. Furthermore, the publisher ensures that the text paper and cover board used have met acceptable environment accrediation standards.

Contents

Foreword	ix
Preface	xi
Introduction	1
A brief history	4
Aims	5
How to Plan a Meta-Analysis	7
Defining the outcomes	8
Choosing the characteristics of the trials that one wants to select	8
The 'grey literature'	9
Finding and evaluating the articles	10
Statistical procedures	13
Interpretation of results	14
Bias in Meta-Analytical Research	15
Sampling bias	16
Selection bias	18
Within study bias	19
Other biases	19
Appendix	20
Statistical Procedures	23
Fixed effects models	24
Random effects models	29

Working Procedures	33
Accuracy of the data	34
Evaluation of the numeric output for each trial	35
Evaluation of the pooled effect	38
Additional considerations on heterogeneity	39
Quantifying heterogeneity: the I^2 index	42
Tests for publication bias	42
Number needed to treat (NNT)	43
Graphical representation	44

How to Read, Evaluate and Present a Meta-Analysis	57
How to read and evaluate a meta-analysis	58
How to present a meta-analysis	59
Examples	61

How to Use the Program	63
General information	64
Installation of the program	64
Structure of the program	65
Use of the program	69
Getting started	70

| References | 87 |

| Glossary | 89 |

| Index | 93 |

Foreword

In their current medical practice, physicians need to be updated with the results of the most important clinical studies. In addition, they are often asked to be part of trials and to evaluate the results of new diagnostic tools and experimental data. A good knowledge of principles and the methodology of statistics is therefore mandatory for all physicians.

Although there has been an increasing interest in evidence-based practice of medicine in the past few years, the data interpretation is still performed badly and statistics are often misused. Among the principal reasons for this is the lack of knowledge concerning the use of mathematical and statistical tools, and a consequent tendency to avoid them if possible. Thus, those physicians who are more familiar with this type of statistics, and who know what is required in good medical practice and how to communicate with their colleagues, are of great help.

This guide to meta-analysis, together with the included statistical software, is the work of a clinician and it deals with the difficulties mentioned above.

The reader is introduced to the principal aspects of meta-analysis using a simple terminology, which does not imply a superficial approach. The most common errors encountered in the practical application of statistical procedures are discussed. The program is designed for easy use, which will help clinicians to utilize meta-analysis. The handbook contains a short section dedicated to the statistical procedures applied. A basic knowledge of statistical methods is an essential starting point, but this manual can also be of great interest and provide useful information for those who have greater experience and are consolidating their statistical knowledge. It is therefore logical that the author's choice has been to concentrate on practical guidelines rather than describing statistical methods.

I am therefore very pleased to write a Foreword for this handbook of meta-analysis, with certainty that it will be a success.

Professor Giuseppe Gallus
Head of the Institute of Medical Statistics
University of Milan, Italy

Preface

The aim of this handbook is to provide the clinical researcher, who is traditionally not familiar with mathematics and statistics, with the basic principles necessary to understand the power of meta-analysis and the essential instruments to perform a good clinical study. For this purpose I have chosen simple and direct language, using easy concepts and examples to enable an intuitive understanding of the problems, at the same time trying to avoid over-simplification.

For these reasons this manual is not intended as a textbook on meta-analysis, but rather a learning tool or a guide for the clinical researcher to understand the basic principles of statistics so that later it may be helpful for correct use of meta-analysis.

This book should enable the reader to perform a meta-analysis, report its results in the correct way and also help understand and critically evaluate meta-analysis published in scientific journals. For further information the reader is referred to other texts or articles.

The software included is easy to use and it contains innovative functions (i.e. moving information from program to program in Windows), additional procedures (cumulative meta-analysis, number needed to treat (NNT), publication bias assessment, test for asymmetry of funnel plot) and graphics not available in other programs (Galbraith's plots, funnel plot and its test for asymmetry). The plot for the sub-group analysis, especially for sensitivity analysis, allows a better understanding of the effect of therapies or procedures on sub-groups in clinical trials. These features make the program a complete and useful tool.

The chapter on statistical analysis explains the computational methods in detail using simple terms and examples. The expert reader will find in this section the formal aspects of the statistical procedure used, whereas a beginner will learn several concepts which will be very useful in understanding meta-analysis.

A complete section is devoted to step-by-step working characteristics of the meta-analysis, which may be useful to the reader to resolve two key questions: "What can we do?" and "How can we do it?" This section reconsiders all the topics previously discussed and uses them in realistic settings by showing in detail the practical applications of NNT, cumulative meta-analysis, publication bias assessment, test for heterogeneity, fixed effect model and random effect model, and so on.

This manual is therefore a theoretical and practical learning tool in its own right, and can be used even without the accompanying software.

Gioacchino Leandro

CHAPTER 1

Introduction

The use of meta-analysis in medicine has increased in recent years due to a growing interest from both physicians and statisticians.

A meta-analysis combines in a single conclusion the results of different studies conducted on the same topic and with the same methods.

Meta-analysis is a tool that helps in understanding the results of intervention in medicine. However, it is not the only or not always the best tool.

The publication of medical reviews and guidelines for good clinical practice has become a common and useful tool for updating most clinical topics. This reflects a need for clinicians to practice 'evidence-based medicine'.

Evidence-based medicine has introduced well-defined rules for the critical evaluation of medical data. The use of meta-analysis has a prominent role in the validation and interpretation of the results of clinical studies. In other words, if a well designed and well conducted meta-analysis has shown that drug A is more effective than drug B, we can assume that this information is correct and there would be no need for further investigation on this issue.

Reporting results of a research protocol is crucial in the process of learning, because it serves both as a conclusion and a new beginning for further study. In fact, a clinical trial is the application of theory to practice, accomplished through well-defined rules of experimentation in order to validate the underlying hypothesis and to achieve relevant results. These results then form the basis for further theories and thus for other clinical trials. Medical practice is greatly influenced by the results of clinical studies, especially if they are brought to public attention through prestigious scientific journals or the mass media.

In the scientific world, new therapies have a greater impact, so a greater number of publications are therefore produced. However, it is hard to define the quality and the importance of each study. Different studies on the same topic often provide discordant conclusions, giving the reader a confused message. In order to clarify the matter we need the help of experts who can provide a conclusive synthesis of the results of different studies.

The growing number of invited reviews and the 'state-of-the-art' lectures is a clear example of the need for unequivocal communication for highly debated topics.

Meta-analysis, when well designed and appropriately performed, is a powerful tool for synthesis. It is an analytical method where both independent and different studies are integrated and their results pooled into a single common result. The meta-analysis, when compared to other forms of reviewing separate studies, has the great advantage of being less influenced by the personal opinion of the reviewer, and provides unbiased conclusions. Moreover, in a meta-analysis all the results of the single studies examined are reported, and the reader may easily recalculate the data and compare them with the conclusions derived by the authors.

The term meta-analysis was coined in 1976. This identifies a process of analysis retrospectively performed on available published data on a specific topic.

When the analysis is done on individual data, it is called a meta-analysis of individual patients. Basically, once the analyst has chosen the most relevant published trials on a subject, instead of performing the meta-analysis on them, he may directly contact the authors of the studies in order to obtain the complete data of the individuals enrolled in the trials. A new set of data is thus created that contains all or part of the information regarding the subjects considered. Meta-analysis of individual patients has techniques of evaluation and objectives different from those explained in this textbook and will not be considered here.

It is a common mistake to consider meta-analysis as a simple statistical test. In fact, meta-analysis is a field of study in itself, and it is important to know about, understand and apply it in all its necessary steps in order to avoid bias. This systematic approach produces results that are worth the effort.

A systematic review as a meta-analysis of the published data is very useful, since a large amount of data is published every year in scientific literature. In 1940 there were roughly 2300 biomedical journals and the number has increased to more than 23000 in 1990, with an incredible quantity of peer-reviewed papers, comments and letters. This large amount of information often contains scattered data and discordant conclusions. Critical works of synthesis with systematic reviews are therefore mandatory.

A correct systematic review on a topic requires collection and analysis of *all* published data and not only of those which are more interesting, relevant, or easily available.

Two steps are thus important for the analysis: first, a complete *collection* of the published literature, and second, the *synthesis* of the information acquired. Such synthesis can be done by an expert in the field as a traditional review, which may have a personal bias, or the synthesis can be made in a more structured and objective fashion using meta-analysis.

The importance of a single study is the result of both its place within the spectrum of a specific topic and the amount of information that it brings to this spectrum. Each study has its intrinsic characteristics and the conclusions it provides may not be generalisable or comparable with those from other studies. On the other hand, some other studies may have similar designs and their results may be taken together for more general considerations. Therefore, adequate attention should be paid to know how the information is obtained from each study to make sure it is correct and can be used appropriately within a meta-analysis.

Systematic reviews and meta-analysis make it possible to validate the results of single studies. This has been the case for several pharmacological intervention studies, where meta-analysis has contributed to establish the role

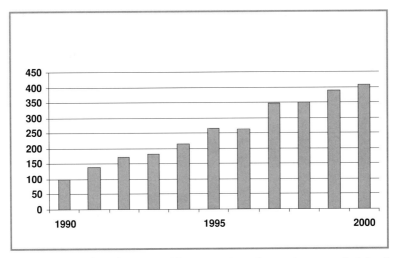

Figure 1.1 Number of articles, grouped by years, where the word meta-analysis has been cited in the abstract.

of a specific drug in the treatment of some diseases, resolving any possible doubt that a single study might have advanced. Moreover, performing a systematic review on a topic requires the critical examination of the methods utilized in the different studies for the evaluation of the data; this may be useful to identify methodological faults in the planning or carrying out of these clinical studies, improving the quality of the research for future.

The interest in meta-analysis and its application in the biomedical world is growing rapidly. A simple search through the Medline system has confirmed the increasing diffusion of this method of analysis. Figure 1.1 shows the number of articles, grouped by years, where the word meta-analysis has been cited in the abstract, implying the use of it in the analysis of the data presented.

This clearly shows that:
- the diffusion of meta-analysis is steadily increasing in the world of biomedical research;
- biomedical journals give importance to articles using meta-analysis.

In summary, knowing how to read, understand, have a critical opinion, and possibly perform, a meta-analysis will be a valuable tool for the researcher who wants to be abreast of modern biomedical research.

A BRIEF HISTORY

The first meta-analysis is attributed to Pearson (1904) who analysed the data from five studies on the correlation between the vaccination for enteritic fever and its mortality.

In 1932 Fisher noticed that the natural logarithm of the value given by the p of a test multiplied by -2 is exactly distributed as a chi-square with two degrees of freedom. From this we can deduce that the sum of m logarithms of p is distributed as a chi-square with $2m$ degrees of freedom:

$$\chi^2_{2m} = -2 \sum_{j=1}^{m} \text{Ln}(p_j)$$

By this means, Fisher identified a way to derive a single p value from the p values of more than one study.

This method is known as *Fisher's inverse chi-squared method*. It was the first of a long series of methods aimed at giving a cumulative value of p.

This type of meta-analysis can be applied to studies where the value p is present without a measure of the effect, or when the design of different studies or the types of treatment are so different that to evaluate a cumulative effect would not be correct.

The limitations of this method are:
1 The values of different studies are not weighted according to their characteristics (e.g. number of subjects, variability.).
2 It is not possible to have an idea of the size of the effect: the p value suggests only the probability for an event to occur by chance without providing any information on the size of the event and therefore on the clinical relevance of the observation.
3 It is impossible to pool studies which have opposite outcomes, in other words if we are evaluating the efficacy of two different procedures, A and B, and one study shows that A is better than B and the other shows that B is better than A, we cannot combine the two studies together because the result may be misleading.
4 It is not possible to further assess the differences, because only the p value is considered without any evaluation of the quality and the methodology of the studies considered.

In 1976, Glass characterised meta-analysis as a specific technique for the first time.

AIMS

One of the main objectives of clinical research is to obtain clear and reliable results that can be utilised in the management of patients and possibly as a basis for clinical guidelines. Clinical trials do not always reach this target and often give contrasting results. Meta-analysis, if correctly used, contributes to achieve this target, and allows for a critical evaluation of the studies under consideration.

Meta-analysis contributes to many aspects of clinical research, for example:
- increases the statistical power of a comparison;
- improves the estimation of the effect of a treatment;
- combines the results of studies that are contrasting;
- answers new questions;
- analyses sub-groups of subjects selected from different studies;
- analyses trends (e.g. within a time-frame, in a sub-group of patients with the same characteristics);
- defines areas in which further studies are needed;
- analyses if and how previous studies have modified knowledge on a certain topic

All these aspects can be evaluated using a methodology, which is intrinsically an objective one as opposed to the 'experts opinion', which is, by definition, subjective.

Moreover, it is always possible to update a meta-analysis if it is 'not conclusive' when new studies are published in the literature.

CHAPTER 2

How to Plan a Meta-Analysis
The Study Design

Meta-analysis is a fundamental part of the process of conducting a systematic review of the literature.

It requires a close collaboration between experts of the topic under investigation and experts in statistical methods applied to the biomedical field.

For the purpose of teaching we can identify different steps in putting together a meta-analysis. Every step has its precise rules aimed at avoiding bias in the analysis to provide more reliable results with an accurate estimation of the events under investigation.

As is the case of a clinical trial, a systematic review must be carefully designed in order to avoid the possibility of biases and errors that may affect the results. It is therefore necessary to define the aims of the analysis and the rules and methods that are necessary to achieve them.

DEFINING THE OUTCOMES

The first step to consider is to define the outcomes to be analysed by meta-analysis. It is advisable to determine a primary outcome (i.e. mortality, efficacy of a treatment) that is considered in all the studies selected for the analysis, and then one or more secondary outcomes that may be useful to answer specific questions (i.e. side effects, sub-groups of patients) that are not necessarily considered in all the studies selected.

CHOOSING THE CHARACTERISTICS OF THE TRIALS THAT ONE WANTS TO SELECT

For this step, it is advisable to consider the largest possible number of studies, and only in a second phase to select studies based on different discriminating factors (number of subjects considered, drop-out rate, randomisation criteria, and so on).

It is important to define where and how the search will be conducted. The most accurate medical bibliographic sources are Medline and Embase. Searching for a topic in only one of the two databases is likely to retrieve only about one third of the published papers and therefore both databases should be used in order to obtain an accurate reference list. In practice, this happens rarely because Medline is a free Web site and easy to use, whereas Embase is a subscription Web site and may be somewhat difficult to use. Although time consuming, alternative options might be to hand-search for published papers, for example in the Index Medicus, and to seek advice from leading experts in the field.

In order to search effectively, it is crucial to choose the correct key words that will precisely identify the topic of our investigation. Usually only studies published in English are considered. Although this is a reasonable choice, sometimes it may be quite restrictive. In fact, some biomedical areas or clinical procedures might be confined to non-English-speaking countries, i.e. 'natural medicine' in China or hyperbaric therapy in Russia.

Once the search has been completed, it is also advisable to check the references cited in each article and to start new searches on that basis.

It may be useful to have two different people conducting the same search: one operating through a computer-based database (i.e. Medline), while the other utilizes more traditional systems, i.e. the Index Medicus, and then exploring the queries through the references cited in the articles found.

When the search is complete, an estimation of the number of papers not found through the two systems should be done (see the Appendix, page 20).

If a more advanced search is needed (i.e. articles published before a specific year or considering only a number of subjects greater than a defined number), the inclusion criteria for the analysis should be decided at the beginning and should be well defined in the study design, explaining the reasons for the selection.

This complete procedure should be described in detail as it represents a fundamental part of the methods section that will be included in the final paper.

THE 'GREY LITERATURE'

> The grey literature is that produced by government, universities, business, and industries, both in print and electronic formats, but which is not controlled by commercial publishing interests and where publishing is not the primary activity of the organization.
> *IIIrd International Conference on Grey Literature, 1997*

Most of the grey literature of biomedical interest is represented by conference and congress proceedings, newsletters, theses, house journals, committee reports and more. However, the most important and easily accessible source for pooling data for meta-analysis is from published abstracts and reports from scientific meetings. Before including data in the meta-analytic process, the following two aspects should be carefully considered:

1. *Data reliability.* Abstracts often report only partial results and they are presented at several congress proceedings. Furthermore, methods and side effects are not always well reported. This problem may be solved by a careful assessment of the reported data in order to avoid duplication of included patients.
2. *Publication bias.* Randomised Controlled Trials (RCTs) presented at scientific meetings are not always published in journals included in reference

databases. It is known that more than one half of the abstracts are published within 2 years and that another one third are under review for publication. It has been estimated that only 16% of them are not traced. The time lag between the conference presentation and the full-text publication may vary, ranging from 1 to 5 years with a median time of 2.7 years. Moreover, papers with significant versus not significant results, and presented (oral presentations) versus not presented papers are published earlier.

In general, we suggest:
- to extend a bibliographic search to abstracts presented at top scientific events in the field of interest;
- to limit the abstract search to within 3–5 years;
- to carefully evaluate the abstracts in order to avoid duplication of included patients;
- to perform the meta-analysis by including and excluding the abstracts to evaluate if and how the pooled effect is modified (sensitivity analysis that is easily run by means of the sub-group analysis option).

FINDING AND EVALUATING THE ARTICLES

It is now easier to find the articles as most of the scientific journals are available on-line. It is, however, far more difficult to read, evaluate and draw the necessary data for the analyses.

A careful reading of all the articles is mandatory. Adequate attention should be paid to identify articles based on the same group of patients, or using sub-groups of subjects already considered in other studies. The inclusion in the analysis of groups of subjects who are not independent will lead to a selection bias (we will discuss this in detail in the following chapter).

There are different ways of reading a scientific paper: a quick and informal reading of the title and the abstract, which can identify key points for further consideration; a more careful reading, which can utilize a scoring system or a check list; and a formal reading with a mathematical check of the data presented. Every reader has his or her own approach to the scientific publication, depending on the experience and the level of information that one wants to obtain from it. However, if one needs to perform a meta-analysis, a formal and careful reading is required in order to gather different aspects that may be helpful to understand the result of the analysis, identify the diversity of the studies considered and explain particular aspects that may emerge from the analysis.

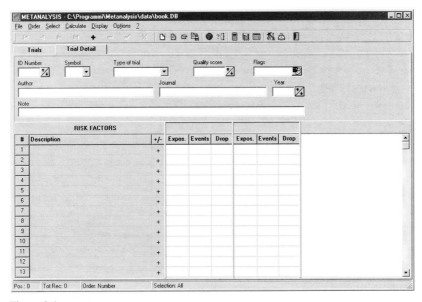

Figure 2.1

Independent of the result that may be obtained, a meta-analysis is also a unique learning experience: the articles will be read several times while the results of the analysis reveal new insights that might have been underestimated on first reading, appreciate skills and tricks of the scientific language, discover what is hidden between the lines and what may not be reported deliberately by the authors in order to avoid possible discrepancies in the results. In other words, one learns a great deal about how to read and how to write a scientific article.

The reading of the selected articles should follow a scheme that will be useful in the collection of the data necessary for the meta-analysis. Figure 2.1 shows an example of a computer-based form for the collection of the data designed for meta-analysis. The form is a computer sheet for data entry in the program of meta-analysis used in the software of this manual.

Specifically, the following information should be entered:

a) *Generic information*: The information about the name of the first author, year, name of the journal and category of publication (peer-reviewed paper or abstract) makes the paper easy to retrieve if further evaluation is needed. The number of the trial (that will appear in all the outputs, either numeric or graphic) should be a progressive number or the reference number of the article included in the bibliography once the meta-analysis is complete and the paper is written.

b) *Design of the trial*: The design information, such as double blinded, open trial, randomised, follow-up period, and all other characteristics of the design, is considered important to understand in detail the different modalities of the studies. The collection of this information should be very careful and precise, because very often the differences in the study design may be a cause of differences and discrepancies in the results.
c) *Treatment of the study group and control group*: A trial is a comparison between two treatments, such as a drug versus a placebo or a new drug versus an old one. Moreover, it is important to register the dosage used in the studies and the length of treatment. Again, differences in the dosage or length of treatment, or the drug used as a control, may generate discrepancies.
d) The number of events, the number of patients at risk in the two groups, and the different *outcomes* are the basis of the calculation used in the meta-analysis. It is important to collect the number of dropouts in different studies (separately for each of the different outcomes) in order to conduct both a 'per protocol' analysis (PP) and a meta-analysis with more selected criteria, considering the dropouts as treatment failures 'intention-to-treat analysis' (ITT). In this case the type of event under analysis (success or failure) will determine how the position of the dropouts are considered: either with the number of events or with the number of subjects treated.
e) The *quality score* is a way of rating the quality of the studies to be included in the meta-analysis, verifying the presence of some 'markers of quality' defined before starting the evaluation procedure. For example, a double-blinded study would be rated 2, a single-blinded 1, and so on. Different scoring systems have been proposed by various authors, each one presenting some advantages and therefore there is no standard system of evaluation available. The discussion of these systems is beyond the scope of this handbook, but we need to consider that:
   - although a score system may be utilized in a meta-analysis, it is preferable to avoid this because firstly there is no general agreement on a standard evaluation system and secondly its use would introduce another bias that needs to be considered;
   - if we use a scoring system, we should divide the studies considered according to its classification in different sub-groups (i.e. low, medium and high quality) and then proceed with a sensitivity analysis (sub-group analysis) in order to verify if the effect of the treatment is variable among the different sub-groups; this use of a scoring system is more acceptable.

In conclusion, we would like to point out that a meta-analysis is by definition already able to evaluate the quality of the studies (we will come back to this later) in a precise and unbiased way. The use of a scoring system that inevitably rejects the small studies in favour of the large studies would lead to the underestimation of the results of some studies and the overestimation of others.

f) *Flags*: it is useful to assign some flags to every trial to identify them for particular characteristics in order to perform an analysis of sensitivity (sub-groups analysis). For example, if we are evaluating all the studies on gastric carcinoma from different geographic areas, the various trials could be segregated based on different risk of gastric cancer in the general population of these areas (low and high risk areas) and a sub-group analysis performed to evaluate if the risk factor under analysis (e.g. *Helicobacter pylori* infection) has a different influence in different areas. Multiple flags may be assigned to a single study to characterise it for multiple factors (i.e. children, high risk areas, non-randomised trials). In this way, we may perform multiple sub-group analyses without much difficulty, or further meta-analysis based only on a portion of the collected studies (e.g. only on children, randomised trials).

STATISTICAL PROCEDURES

The statistical methods will be described in detail in Chapter 4. This handbook will explain how to choose a proper method . These procedures will be described briefly in this section giving a few insights that will be developed later.

The results of a trial may be expressed as odds ratio (OR) or risk difference (RD), which is also known in epidemiology as absolute risk reduction (ARR). As meta-analysis is a way of aggregating the results of multiple trials, the results obtained may be expressed as *pooled odds ratio* (ORp) or *pooled risk difference* (RDp).

In order to pool the results of the different studies, we should assume that these results would give an evaluation of effect, which would be the same for all studies, and that the effects evaluated would be part of the same distribution (sample estimates of the same mean). This assumption should be verified with a statistical test, the *test for heterogeneity*. If this is correct, in a further analysis we can use formulas based on this assumption, called *fixed effects models*. If we are not constrained by the studies belonging to the same population (i.e. the studies evaluated are sampled from a population that contains several populations, each with its own mean), and therefore we assume that the variability of the results depends on the variability of the intra- and inter-studies, we will use procedures called *random effects models*.

Other statistical procedures are the *test for publication bias*, the *number needed to treat* (NNT) and the *cumulative meta-analysis*, which will be discussed in the following chapters.

INTERPRETATION OF RESULTS

The interpretation of the results obtained with a meta-analysis is the result of a series of evaluations that start from the evaluation of the size of the pooled effect, the possible causes of heterogeneity, the evaluation of the 'stability' of the meta-analysis (i.e. the pooled effect is not changed significantly by the addition of new studies), and the calculation of the number needed to be treated.

These topics will be covered in the chapter on 'working procedures' of this handbook (see Chapter 5), since for the clinical researcher a practical approach with examples is far more useful than a theoretical one.

CHAPTER 3

Bias in Meta-Analytical Research

These are several biases that may alter the results of a meta-analysis.

Knowing the possible biases, it is essential to avoid them or at least to minimize their effects.

There are multiple biases that may influence the results of a meta-analysis. Amongst them, the researcher usually only considers the publication bias, while all the others are generally underestimated or ignored.

In this chapter we will list all the possible biases and give some advice on how to avoid them.

SAMPLING BIAS

This bias is caused by the difficulties in retrieving all the studies on a topic.

1 *Publication bias*: Since usually only studies where a significant difference is found are published, this implies that some completed studies are not published and therefore cannot be considered in the meta-analysis. These may have results discordant from the published studies. Therefore, the meta-analysis might have had a different result if all trials could have been considered. However, quite often non-published studies are presented as abstracts for scientific meetings and therefore we can have a more comprehensive analysis by also including the abstracts.

The publication bias has two forms. The *conformity publication bias* is due to the fact that, if there is a common opinion already established on a topic, it will be easier to publish studies that are in accord with this opinion, while discordant results are less likely to be accepted.

The opposite of this 'editorial philosophy' is the *inverse conformity publication bias*, where papers confirming already established data may be considered redundant, while discordant results may be accepted as a novelty.

The publication bias has three different sources: the author, the sponsor of the trial, and the editorial policy of the journal to which the paper has been submitted.

Both authors and the editorial boards of journals are usually less interested in publishing a paper with negative results. The *sponsor* of the study is not usually happy with results that do not confirm the efficacy of a new medicine or intervention.

There are several ways to evaluate the presence and the importance of a publication bias, since its effects cannot be eliminated. Among them, the more commonly used are:

(a) The graphic method by Light and Pillemer (*Funnel Plot*) for which a plot is calculated using the effect size and the sample size of every trial: the resulting figure, in the absence of publication bias, is a reversed funnel. Some alternatives for X and Y axes are available. The X axis may represent Risk Ratio, Odds Ratio and Risk Difference. The Y axis may

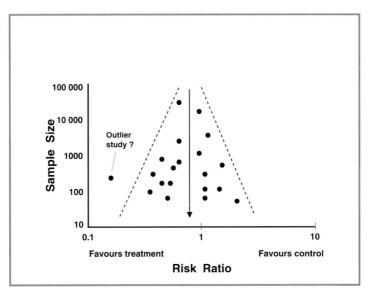

Figure 3.1

represent the trial size, the precision of the trial (1/SE), the variance and a number of other options. The standard representation is given by the Odds Ratio and the trial size. Other representations have particular aims that go beyond the purpose of this work. This is a very approximate method since it is only a visual judgment of the data. It is used very commonly because it is easy to complete and gives a simple figure. Its use is acceptable only if the meta-analysis includes a large number of studies but not in a meta-analysis with a small number of studies. A good practice to avoid evaluating the publication bias only according to visual judgment is to use a test for asymmetry applied to the funnel plot. We will discuss later the test for asymmetry.

(b) Klein's method is based on the following hypothesis: if the unpublished studies have the same characteristics, with regard to the number of subjects and their variability as the published ones, how many unpublished studies with negative or null results are needed to influence the results of the meta-analysis? This number is the whole number immediately above:

$$\left(\frac{k \, \text{Ln} \, OR}{1.96}\right)^2 \overline{W} - k$$

where $\overline{W}$ is the mean of the weights of k trials per $W_i = \frac{1}{V_i}$ (see page 42 for details).

This test does not exactly answer the question 'is there or not a publication bias?'. It is instead an indirect test of reliability of the meta-analysis when it is dealing with problems of publication bias. Furthermore, a quantitative approach is to be preferred and the META program will provide this assessment which is the Publication Bias Assessment.

2 If the search is internet based (e.g. Medline), there are other kinds of biases:
  2.1 *Indexing bias*: This occurs due to poor indexing of the studies in the internet database. This error may especially occur when an article is new and it has been introduced into the database recently. In a second phase, checks are made and the mistakes are usually corrected.
  2.2 *Search bias*: This occurs due to difficulties in retrieving all the indexed papers in the database. The rate of studies identified by an expert user utilizing the internet-based databases is between 32% and 80%, and it is far lower with inexperienced users. For this reason, it is crucial to pay attention to the search strategy. It is always useful to invite several people to conduct independent searches and then compare their results.
3 If the search is based both on internet-based databases and on non-internet-based methods (review of the literature, etc.) there are other biases:
  3.1 *Reference bias*: This occurs when there is a likelihood that some studies are cited frequently and others may not be cited at all.
  3.2 *Multiple publication bias*: This occurs due to the publication of the same results in multiple articles.
  3.3 *Multiply-used subjects bias*: This occurs due to publication of results involving different sub-groups derived from the same group of subjects.

All these biases can be avoided by a careful reading of the articles.

SELECTION BIAS

1 *Inclusion criteria bias*: This may occur if the inclusion criteria decided for use in the meta-analysis somehow exclude relevant studies. Since it is an inclusion bias, this error is difficult to detect, quantify and avoid once the criteria have been selected.
2 *Selector bias*: If precise criteria of selection are not defined from the beginning, the person involved in the search may use his or her own criteria

and this may give varying results. An ideal way to avoid this bias is to define precise selection criteria and evaluate the studies according to the criteria without considering their results.

WITHIN STUDY BIAS

Once the papers have been selected, there may be difficulties obtaining the data we need from the results of the studies.
1 *Bias caused by the meta-analyst:*
   1.1 *Extractor bias*: This occurs due to inaccuracy in the recording of the results. This is very common and difficult to avoid. It may greatly affect the result of the analysis. It is always useful to perform two separate readings and to resolve discordant evaluations.
   1.2 *Quality score bias*: If the system used to score the quality of the papers is not strictly defined, there is the possibility of a personal judgment by the reader that may affect the results of the analysis. The bias is easily avoidable by not using any scoring system.
2 *Bias due to inadequate accuracy in reporting the results by the authors of the studies:*
   2.1 *Reporting bias*: An example of this bias is a trial designed to evaluate multiple outcomes, but where only the significant results are reported. This bias is unavoidable and often impossible to quantify. One can always contact the authors to obtain all the results. Very often having unreported data in a study means that the study is of poor quality.
   2.2 *Recording error bias*: It is due to errors made by the authors interpreting the results obtained. It occurs in about 1% of the data reported. It is not very important in a meta-analysis, because it is a random error, especially if the number of subjects is large enough. It adds only an element of imprecision to the estimate.

OTHER BIASES

These are not considered often; however, they may be as important as those listed above.
1 *Geographical bias*: It may not be advisable to group the results of studies conducted in different geographical areas, because the differences in prevalence and incidence of pathologies and risk factors may have important effects on the results. If this is the case, it may be inappropriate to do a meta-analysis on all the studies in order to obtain an estimate of

the mean effect. Instead, a sensitivity analysis should be performed evaluating sub-groups of studies from the same area and subsequently decide whether all of the results can be pooled together.
2 *Follow-up time bias*: The length of the follow-up is relevant if there is a time-dependent effect in the outcome considered. Studies using the same drug at the same dosage may have different results if the drug has been administered for different periods of time. If the time-dependent effect is not considered, and it is a very common issue in the clinical setting, the evaluation of the mean effect can be biased.

APPENDIX

In this appendix an interesting technique for the evaluation of the completeness of the search for references is described. It allows an acceptable evaluation of the number of papers that have not been found despite the two different methods utilized and previously described. This is very important information for the correct evaluation of a meta-analysis.

This system is an application of the 'capture–mark–recapture' method used by biologists in order to count the whole number of a single animal species in a geographic area. If, for example, we want to know the number of sharks in the Mediterranean Sea, we can mark all the sharks that we are able to catch and then release them in a defined period of time. After a period of time necessary for the marked sharks to get dispersed in the sea, we count the prevalence of the marked sharks among all the sharks caught in a defined period of time: this will give us an estimate of the total number of sharks in the area.

		Database		
		Yes	No	
Hand-search	Yes	M	$n - m$	n
	No	$M - m$	?	$N - n$
		M	$N - M$	N

In our case, let us assume that the Medline-based search for papers on a particular topic in a defined period of time has given a total of M papers, while the search based on the Index Medicus and the references of other papers has resulted in a number of n papers. Of all those, a number m of papers would be included in both groups of papers. We can now build the table shown.

Considering the formulas for the calculation of the expected value, N, the total number of papers (found + not found), assuming the independence of the sources, will be:

$N = M(n/m)$

This estimate of maximum likelihood is partially distorted for small numbers, and it could be more precisely obtained using the Chapman method:

$N = (M+1)(n+1)/(m+1) - 1$

The variance of N will be:

$\mathrm{Var}(N) = (M+1)(n+1)(M-m)(n-m)/[(m+1)2(m+2)]$

with a confidence interval of 95%.

A mandatory requirement for the use of the capture and recapture method is the independence of the sources.

CHAPTER 4
Statistical Procedures

Knowing the statistical procedures is of great importance in choosing which test is needed and why.

Different results with different software packages are the result of different approximation methods used in the software formulae.

This chapter contains several formulae which could be very helpful to those who want to understand the calculations used in the procedures. This chapter is also useful in understanding meta-analysis in general as it contains fundamental elements and concepts of meta-analysis.

As stated earlier, meta-analysis is a procedure that allows aggregation of the results of multiple studies. This aggregation is not the simple sum of the data obtained from all the studies, but a procedure that "weights" the results of each study according to its precision. In fact, if the precision is estimated on the width of the dispersion, namely the variance, then the weight of each study i is given by the inverse of the variance:

$$W_i = \frac{1}{V_i} \tag{1}$$

where W_i is the weight and V_i the variance of the outcome of the study.

In other words, if a study has a wide variance (= dispersion = imprecision) it will have a small weight in determining the final result of the analysis (the "pooled" result of the meta-analysis), while a study with a small variance (= greater precision) will have a greater weight.

The general formula of the meta-analysis expresses the global outcome D in terms of a weighted mean:

$$D = \frac{\sum w_i d_i}{\sum w_i} \tag{2}$$

with the sum extended to n studies.

The numerator is an expression of the above-mentioned concept, the denominator has the simple function of normalizing the weight used.

Once it is established that the measure of the outcome of each single study is to be weighted by its precision, one has to define what needs to be evaluated in the study, or the d_i of formula (2).

This entity could be either the difference in the rate of the event between the two groups under study or the Odds Ratio (OR).

The procedures used in the calculation may be divided into two categories: fixed effects models and random effects models.

FIXED EFFECTS MODELS

The fixed effects models are based on the assumption that the available studies taken as a group give an estimate of the same treatment effect so that the estimated effects can be considered as part of the same distribution (sample estimates of the same mean). However, this hypothesis needs to be proven using a statistical procedure named "test for heterogeneity".

This analysis allows the investigator to assess whether the studies under evaluation deal with the same parameter or not.

The test for heterogeneity is based on the following equation:

$$\chi^2 = \sum_{j=1}^{m} w_j \left(\hat{\Theta}_j - \hat{\Theta}\right)^2 \qquad (3)$$

In the case where the null hypothesis of homogeneity is satisfied, the above equation approximately distributes as a chi-square with $m-1$ degree of freedom. Here $\hat{\Theta}_j$ is the estimate of the effect in the $j-n$ study, $\hat{\Theta}$ is the estimate of the pooled effect and w_j is the weight of the $j-n$ study.

The results of such analysis can be represented as a table as follows:

Studied condition (e.g. ulcer healing)

	Yes	No	Total
Drug N	A	B	A + B
Drug S	C	D	C + D
Total	A + C	B + D	

A + B is the total number of individuals treated with the drug under study (new drug), A is the number of subjects included in the group where the event (i.e. healing) has occurred and B is the group of patients where the expected effect did not occur. C + D is the number of subjects treated according to a current standard of care (standard drug), C is the number of subjects included in the group where the event occurred and D is the group of patients where the expected effect did not occur.

The calculation of the *difference of percentage* (also called absolute risk reduction (ARR)) is not a difficult computational problem and is performed by applying the following formula:

$$d = \frac{A}{A+B} - \frac{C}{C+D} \qquad (4)$$

or the more general formula:

$$d = \frac{O_i}{N_i} - \frac{O_s}{N_s} \qquad (4b)$$

where O is the observed events (deaths, complications, etc.), N is the number of subjects included in the study, i is the new treatment and s is the standard treatment.

The 95% confidence interval is calculated by the usual formula:

$$CI(95\%) = d \pm 1.96 * SE(d) \tag{5}$$

where d is the percentage difference and $SE(d)$ is the standard error of the difference calculated according to the following formula:

$$SE(d) = \sqrt{\frac{O_s * (N_s - O_s)}{N_s^3} - \frac{O_i * (N_i - O_i)}{N_i^3}} \tag{6}$$

After having calculated the difference and the standard error of the difference in each study, the pooled effect is obtained by applying the general formula of the meta-analysis (2) and is not to be confused with the D of formula (4). The confidence interval of D is calculated as follows:

$$CI(95\%) = D \pm \frac{1.96}{\sqrt{\sum w_i}} \tag{7}$$

The test for heterogeneity is calculated as follows:

$$\chi^2 = \sum \left[w_i * [d_i - D]^2 \right] \tag{8}$$

where D is the pooled effect, d_i and w_i are the percentage difference and the weight of the $i - n$ study, respectively.

The *Odds Ratio (OR)* needs some further detailed explanation. The calculation of the OR may be performed according to different methods. The most used are the methods by Mantel-Haenszel, Peto, and Gart. Some examples are illustrated step-by-step in order to make them easier to understand.

A) Mantel-Haenszel method

Considering the data included in the table on p. 25, the OR is calculated using the following formula:

$$OR = \frac{A/B}{C/D} = \frac{A * D}{B * C} \tag{9}$$

which defines the result of the comparison within each study.

The OR, especially for rare events, may be considered as an estimate of the Relative Risk, and indicates how many times the exposure (the particular procedure or the treatment) increases the risk of the event. In this case, $A + B \approx B$ and $C + D \approx D$.

By examining formula (9) it is evident that, if the tables include some zeros, the estimate may have a value of 0 or ∞. In order to avoid this problem, in the program a value of 0.5 is always added to every single cell. This may cause very small differences in the results when compared to other software programs.

The 95% confidence interval for the OR can be calculated using the standard formula:

$$CI(95\%) = \exp[\text{Ln OR} \pm 1.96 * SE(\text{Ln OR})] \qquad (10)$$

where SE(Ln OR) is the standard error of the natural logarithm of the OR.

As a practical example, we now consider two studies on lung cancer in women exposed to passive cigarette smoking (Garfinkel et al., 1985, Lam et al., 1987), see Table 4.1.

Table 4.1 Example of studies on lung cancer in women exposed to passive cigarette smoking.

		Exposed	Not exposed	Total
Study 1	Cases	90	44	134
	Controlled	245	157	402
	Total	335	201	536
Study 2	Cases	115	84	199
	Controlled	152	183	335
	Total	267	267	534

Formula (9) allows us to calculate the OR of the two studies:

$$OR_1 = \frac{A * D}{B * C} = \frac{90 * 157}{44 * 245} = 1.31$$

$$OR_2 = \frac{115 * 183}{84 * 152} = 1.65$$

The approximated variance, acceptable when the OR is close to 1, is calculated using the following formula:

$$V_i = \frac{n_i}{(b_i * c_i)} \qquad (11)$$

Then:

$$V_1 = \frac{536}{44 * 245} = 0.05$$

$$V_2 = \frac{534}{84 * 152} = 0.042$$

The weight of each study is calculated from (1):

$$W_1 = \frac{1}{V_1} = \frac{1}{0.05} = 20.00$$

$$W_2 = \frac{1}{V_2} = \frac{1}{0.042} = 23.81$$

The estimate of the pooled OR according to Mantel-Haenszel is obtained by applying formula (2):

$$OR_{M-H} = \frac{(OR_1 * W_1) + (OR_2 * W_2)}{W_1 + W_2} = \frac{1.31 * 20 + 1.65 * 23.81}{23.81 + 20.00} = 1.4$$

The variance of the OR_{M-H} is calculated according to a complicated formula, which in this case gives us the result of 0.019. The estimate of the 95% confidence interval is calculated by applying formula (10), which provides us with the lower and upper limits: 1.14–1.95.

Due to multiple advantages and precision, this method is widely used and is frequently found in computer programs.

B) Peto method

The Peto method is based on a modification of the Mantel-Haenszel method.

The first step is the calculation of the expected value of the events in every single group, according to the standard formula of the product of the marginal totals divided by n. Specifically, considering the table 4.1, we have:

$$E_1 = \frac{(a_1 + b_1) * (a_1 + c_1)}{n_1} = \frac{134 * 335}{536} = 83.75$$

$$E_2 = \frac{(a_2 + b_2) * (a_2 + c_2)}{n_2} = \frac{199 * 267}{534} = 99.5$$

The difference between the observed and expected events is then calculated:

Study 1 = 90 − 83.75 = 6.25

Study 2 = 115 − 99.5 = 15.5

The variance of these quantities is:

$$V_i = \frac{[E_i * (b_i + d_i) * (c_i + d_i)]}{n_i * (n_i - 1)}$$

And then:

Study 1 = (90 ∗ 201 ∗ 402)/(536 ∗ 535) = 25.36

Study 2 = (99.5 ∗ 267 ∗ 335)/(534 ∗ 533) = 31.27

The natural logarithm of the OR_P is calculated:

Ln OR_P = sum of (observed − expected)/sum of the variances

Ln OR_P = $(6.25 + 15.5)/(25.36 + 31.27) = 21.75/56.63 = 0.38$

and:

OR_P = exp(Ln OR_P) = 1.46

The 95% confidence interval is calculated as follows:

$$CI(95\%) = \exp\left(OR_P \pm \frac{1.96}{\sqrt{\sum V_i}}\right)$$

which easily gives us the lower and upper limits: 1.13–1.90.

Using the Peto calculation, the presence of a 0 value in a cell does not affect the calculation, and therefore no approximation is needed.

Tests for heterogeneity

Mantel-Haenszel method:

$$Q = \sum w_i \,(Ln\ OR_i - Ln\ OR_{MH})$$

Peto method:

$$Q = \sum \left[w_i * (O_i - E_i)^2\right] - \frac{\sum (O_i - E_i)^2}{\sum V_i}$$

where Q has a chi-square distribution with degrees of freedom equal to $n - 1$ studies. The statistical power of this test is very low if the meta-analysis includes a few studies, thus the rejection of the hypothesis of heterogeneity is not always a valid test to establish that the same quantity is being measured. In particular, obvious clinical heterogeneity in different studies may not result in statistical heterogeneity. Use of sensitivity analyses may be needed to establish whether clinical differences influence the results of the meta-analysis.

RANDOM EFFECTS MODELS

These models of analysis do not require the assumption that each study is derived from the same population of patients and therefore the n studies can be considered as a part of separate populations, each with their own mean. Therefore, the variability of the estimate may have two sources: within the study and between the studies.

The DerSimonian–Laird method applied to the ORs needs the following calculations:

$$\text{Ln OR}_{dl} = \frac{\sum (w_i^* * \text{Ln OR}_i)}{\sum w_i^*}$$

where

$$w_i^* = \frac{1}{\left[D + \left(\frac{1}{w_i}\right)\right]}$$

$$D = \frac{[Q - (S - 1)] * \sum w_i}{\left[(\sum w_i)^2 - \sum w_i^2\right]}$$

where S is the number of the studies and

$$Q = \sum w_i (\text{Ln OR}_i - \text{Ln OR}_{MH})$$

and

$$\text{variance}_i^* = \sum w_i^*$$

There is no universal consensus on the choice of fixed or random effect models. The next chapter will illustrate in more detail some theoretical controversies regarding this important aspect of meta-analysis.

Quantifying heterogeneity

A detailed theoretical discussion on indices of quantitative evaluation of heterogeneity is beyond the aim of this work.

The three main indicators of the quantitative evaluation of heterogeneity are the following:

> **H** is the square root of the chi-square for heterogeneity statistics divided by its degrees of freedom. It describes the relative excess in Q over its degrees of freedom.
>
> **R** is the ratio of the standard error of the mean from the random effect meta-analysis to the standard error of a fixed effect meta-analytic estimate. It describes the inflation in the confidence interval for a summary estimate under a random effect model compared with a fixed effect model.
>
> **I²** is a transformation of the H that describes the proportion of total variation in study estimate that is due to heterogeneity.

The main characteristics of these indicators, as well as their strengths, are:
- the dependence on the extent of heterogeneity;
- the scale invariance (this feature makes it possible to compare these indicators also from meta-analyses with different scales and outcomes); and
- the size invariance, i.e. these measures are not dependent on the number of the studies.

Quantifying publication bias

The calculation of the intercept and the β-coefficient follows the same procedure as the regression analysis.

$$\alpha = \sum_{i=1}^{n} \frac{y_i}{n} - \beta \sum_{i=1}^{n} \frac{x_i}{n}$$

$$\beta = \frac{\sum_{i=1}^{n}(x_i - \bar{x})(y_i - \bar{y})}{\sum_{i=1}^{n}(x_i - \bar{x})^2}$$

$$SE(\alpha) = \sqrt{\frac{\sum_{i=1}^{n}(y_i - \hat{y})^2}{n-2} * \left(\frac{1}{n-2} + \frac{\bar{x}^2}{\sum(x_i - \bar{x})^2}\right)}$$

for $x = \dfrac{1}{SE(\Delta)}$ and $y = \dfrac{\Delta}{SE(\Delta)}$

$95\% \ CI(\alpha) = \alpha \pm 1.96 * SE(\alpha).$

CHAPTER 5

Working Procedures

The essence of meta-analysis relies on a careful analysis of the data, on the numerical approach, and also on a standard and innovative graphical approach.

The supervision by an expert statistician, or at least the discussion of the results obtained with him or her, is essential for a complete understanding of meta-analysis and a better use of this statistical tool.

The present chapter gives a step-by-step guide through the practical phases of the analysis, illustrating how to deal successfully with problems that may be encountered during the procedure.

The understanding of the following practical instructions as well as allowing one to perform a meta-analysis correctly, will also allow a critical evaluation of a meta-analysis performed by others. In the latter case, it is essential to dissect all the factors that explain how the investigators went about their meta-analysis. As a useful start-up project, one can reproduce a meta-analysis already published following the instructions described below.

After completing the phases of study design, literature search and evaluation of studies under analysis according to the procedures already described, and following completion of the forms for each study, the meta-analysis can be performed and the results interpreted.

ACCURACY OF THE DATA

Once the data are entered and the calculations made, the evaluation of the results can proceed. The output of a meta-analysis must always include the original data, which should be checked for input errors.

The data must always be searched for in the original papers in order to perform an independent analysis and evaluation. The absence of the original data in a report in a meta-analysis always represents a potential error, suggesting that the authors may not want their statistical work to be double-checked by other investigators.

Figure 5.1 shows the data relative to Example 1. These are a series of clinical trials studying the effect of the drug cimetidine on gastric ulcer healing after four weeks of treatment. The papers are ordered by year of publication,

	Author	Journal	Score	Year	PLACEBO Ent.	PLACEBO Obs.	CIMETIDINE Ent.	CIMETIDINE Obs.
1	Bader	Clin Exc Med	0	1977	27	10	26	18
2	Frost	Br Med J	0	1977	22	6	23	18
3	Englert	Gastroenterol	0	1978	62	38	60	42
4	Cremer	Bruss Exec Med	0	1978	11	8	8	7
5	Lambert	Bruss Exc Med	0	1978	25	9	24	17
6	Dick	Gastroenterol	0	1978	29	12	30	18
7	Navert	Gastroenterol	0	1978	10	3	21	10
8	Ciclitira	Gut	0	1979	25	13	35	23
9	Landecker	Med J Austr	0	1979	23	13	25	21
10	Clarke	Austr NZ J Med	0	1980	15	3	15	9
11	Isemberg	New Engl J Med	0	1983	35	9	38	20
12	Dawson	Scand J Gastroenterol	0	1984	20	6	20	11
13	Graham	Ann Int Med	0	1985	67	30	66	43
14	Frank	Clin Ther	0	1989	80	44	83	63
				TOTALS	451	204	474	320

Figure 5.1

which is the standard way of data presentation in the software. A different presentation may be used in selected settings such as the evaluation of a given effect according to the size of the sample, or to the frequency of the event in the control group.

For both groups (treated subjects and controls) there are two columns of data: number of patients studied and the events (healing in this case) observed. To make the reading of the table easier, entering the first group as the controls followed by the study group is recommended.

Having these data available, one can perform and analyse 'per protocol' (PP) or, when needed, by an 'intention-to-treat' analysis (ITT) where the dropouts are taken as failures. In the case of PP, the dropouts are not evaluated in the analysis and the number of such patients will be automatically subtracted from the total number of subjects studied. In the ITT, if the event is favourable (ulcer healing, etc.), the number of subjects is not modified, whereas if the event is adverse (death, ulcer, relapse etc.) the number of dropouts is added to the number of observed events. This procedure is currently used in biomedical research but it has a problem in that the assignment of a subject to the group of observed events is made in a systematic rather than random way, contrary to what it would be in an intention-to-treat procedure.

In the example provided, the data do not include the dropouts and this is justified by the fact that in those years Cimetidine was a great innovation to cure the patients with gastric ulcer, the total number of cases was extremely small and the follow-up very short (four weeks). All the reported studies were original papers with the exception of the abstract by Navert (no.7). Overall, the analysis has been performed with 14 trials, most of them were small in size, with a total of 925 patients, 451 receiving a Placebo and 474 cimetidine.

EVALUATION OF THE NUMERIC OUTPUT FOR EACH TRIAL

The numeric output is evaluated by selecting all the available options in the menu that displays all the options when using the program.

Figure 5.2 shows the 'simplified' output that contains, for each trial, the calculations related to the Risk Difference and to the Odds Ratio, according to Gart and Peto. This is usually more than sufficient in a standard procedure.

In this example, one can see that the single trials have apparently contrasting results: in fact, seven trials show a significant superiority of Cimetidine, while the other seven do not show any difference as compared to the placebo.

	Difference of percentage			CONDENSED GART			PETO		
	Δ	MIN	MAX	OR	MIN	MAX	OR	MIN	MAX
1	32.19	6.77	57.62	3.63	1.19	11.07	3.55	1.22	10.34
2	50.99	25.88	76.10	8.54	2.29	31.81	7.41	2.33	23.61
3	8.71	−8.07	25.49	1.46	0.69	3.08	1.47	0.70	3.09
4	14.77	−20.13	49.67	2.06	0.24	17.68	2.32	0.26	20.42
5	34.83	8.67	61.00	4.05	1.26	13.06	3.94	1.30	11.95
6	18.62	−6.45	43.69	2.07	0.75	5.75	2.08	0.76	5.72
7	17.62	−17.92	53.16	1.96	0.43	8.94	2.01	0.45	9.04
8	13.71	−11.40	38.83	1.74	0.62	4.88	1.75	0.62	4.96
9	27.48	2.64	52.32	3.72	1.02	13.60	3.68	1.07	12.62
10	40.00	7.99	72.01	5.22	1.11	24.58	5.01	1.19	21.06
11	26.92	5.43	48.40	3.09	1.17	8.17	3.03	1.19	7.70
12	25.00	−4.64	54.64	2.70	0.76	9.55	2.71	0.79	9.35
13	20.38	3.82	36.93	2.28	1.14	4.55	2.26	1.15	4.47
14	20.90	6.64	35.17	2.54	1.31	4.93	2.51	1.32	4.79

Figure 5.2

This is evident by considering the 95% confidence interval: if this interval includes one in the OR or zero in the RD, the result is not statistically significant.

However, considering Figure 5.2, the central measure (either the OR or the RD) is always in favour of cimetidine and it is more or less consistent in all the trials considered. This could suggest that the non-significant result may be due to the small number of subjects (i.e. small sample size, low power). A confirmation of this suspicion may be obtained from the results of the meta-analysis.

	Author	Difference of percentage							
		PLACEBO		CIMETIDINE					
		Ent.	%Obs.	Ent.	%Obs.	Δ	ES(Δ)	MIN	MAX
1	Bader	27	37.04	26	69.23	32.19	12.97	6.77	57.62
2	Frost	22	27.27	23	78.26	50.99	12.81	25.88	76.10
3	Englert	62	61.29	60	70.00	8.71	8.56	−8.07	25.49
4	Cremer	11	72.73	8	87.50	14.77	17.81	−20.13	49.67
5	Lambert	25	36.00	24	70.83	34.83	13.35	8.67	61.00
6	Dick	29	41.38	30	60.00	18.62	12.79	−6.45	43.69
7	Navert	10	30.00	21	47.62	17.62	18.13	−17.92	53.16
8	Ciclitira	25	52.00	35	65.71	13.71	12.81	−11.40	38.83
9	Landecker	23	56.52	25	84.00	27.48	12.67	2.64	52.32
10	Clarke	15	20.00	15	60.00	40.00	16.33	7.99	72.01
11	Isemberg	35	25.71	38	52.63	26.92	10.96	5.43	48.40
12	Dawson	20	30.00	20	55.00	25.00	15.12	−4.64	54.64
13	Graham	67	44.78	66	65.15	20.38	8.44	3.82	36.93
14	Frank	80	55.00	83	75.90	20.90	7.28	6.64	35.17

Figure 5.3

ODDS RATIO (Logarithmic scale - GART)									
Author	Y	X	Ln(OR)	ES	Min	Max	OR	MIN	MAX
1 Bader	2.26	1.76	1.29	0.57	0.17	2.40	3.63	1.19	11.07
2 Frost	3.20	1.49	2.14	0.67	0.83	3.46	8.54	2.29	31.81
3 Englert	1.00	2.63	0.38	0.38	−0.36	1.12	1.46	0.69	3.08
4 Cremer	0.66	0.91	0.72	1.10	−1.43	2.87	2.06	0.24	17.68
5 Lambert	2.34	1.68	1.40	0.60	0.23	2.57	4.05	1.26	13.06
6 Dick	1.40	1.92	0.73	0.52	−0.29	1.75	2.07	0.75	5.75
7 Navert	0.87	1.29	0.67	0.78	−0.85	2.19	1.96	0.43	8.94
8 Ciclitira	1.05	1.90	0.55	0.53	−0.48	1.59	1.74	0.62	4.88
9 Landecker	1.98	1.51	1.31	0.66	0.02	2.61	3.72	1.02	13.60
10 Clarke	2.09	1.27	1.65	0.79	0.10	3.20	5.22	1.11	24.58
11 Isemberg	2.28	2.02	1.13	0.50	0.16	2.10	3.09	1.17	8.17
12 Dawson	1.54	1.55	0.99	0.64	−0.27	2.26	2.70	0.76	9.55
13 Graham	2.33	2.83	0.82	0.35	0.13	1.52	2.28	1.14	4.55
14 Frank	2.76	2.96	0.93	0.34	0.27	1.60	2.54	1.31	4.93

Figure 5.4

If a detailed analysis of the calculations performed for obtaining the results showed in Figure 5.2 is needed, this can be done by choosing the option Expanded results. The output will provide the information shown in Figures 5.3–5.5.

Figure 5.3 shows the data relative to the Risk Difference organised in columns showing the patients included and the rate of events (healing) that occurred in the two groups studied (placebo and cimetidine), the difference in rates with their relative standard error and the 95% confidence interval of the risk difference.

ODDS RATIO (Observed-Expected-PETO)										
Author	PLACEBO		CIMETIDINE			O-E	V	OR	Min	Max
	Ent.	Obs.	Ent.	Obs.	Expec.					
1 Bader	27	10	26	18	13.7	4.26	0.297	3.55	1.22	10.34
2 Frost	22	6	23	18	12.3	5.73	0.349	7.41	2.33	23.61
3 Englert	62	38	60	42	39.3	2.66	0.144	1.47	0.70	3.09
4 Cremer	11	8	8	7	6.3	0.68	1.231	2.32	0.26	20.42
5 Lambert	25	9	24	17	12.7	4.27	0.321	3.94	1.30	11.95
6 Dick	29	12	30	18	15.3	2.75	0.257	2.08	0.76	5.72
7 Navert	10	3	21	10	8.8	1.19	0.587	2.01	0.45	9.04
8 Ciclitira	25	13	35	23	21.0	2.00	0.281	1.75	0.62	4.96
9 Landecker	23	13	25	21	17.7	3.29	0.396	3.68	1.07	12.62
10 Clarke	15	3	15	9	6.0	3.00	0.537	5.01	1.19	21.06
11 Isemberg	35	9	38	20	15.1	4.90	0.226	3.03	1.19	7.70
12 Dawson	20	6	20	11	8.5	2.50	0.399	2.71	0.79	9.35
13 Graham	67	30	66	43	36.2	6.77	0.121	2.26	1.15	4.47
14 Frank	80	44	83	63	54.5	8.52	0.108	2.51	1.32	4.79

Figure 5.5

Figure 5.4 shows the calculations of the Odds ratio according to Gart. Figure 5.5 shows the Odds ratio according to Peto. Peto's statistical method is based on the difference between the expected values and those observed in the study, and it is not affected by the presence of cells containing zero as a value.

The expanded output is not required for each meta-analysis as it represents only the details of the calculations performed. It does not add information useful to the analysis. It is designed for those who wish to obtain further information on what has been done and, in particular, to enable a manual check on the statistical procedure.

EVALUATION OF THE POOLED EFFECT

The printed page that shows the summary of the meta-analysis has two distinct parts.

The first shows the analysis performed by the *fixed effects models*. This model requires that the estimates of treatment effect obtained from all trials belong to the same distribution. This requirement has to be verified by some procedures. The first is the Galbraith plot, which will be described in a subsequent chapter. The other procedure is related to the formal test of statistical heterogeneity, which is more precise because it does not have any approximation that is inherent in the graphical representation.

The pooled effect for the data considered in the current example is shown in Figure 5.6.

The result of this test for heterogeneity is indicated by **Q**, which is a chi-square with the degrees of freedom (**df**) shown below it, under the hypothesis of homogeneity. The statistical significance is also shown in the same section (p(Q)). Which of the four tests of statistical heterogeneity is used, is related to the procedure chosen to evaluate the data. This aspect will be discussed later.

Once it is clear that the test for heterogeneity is not significant ($p = 0.584$), the hypothesis that the trials under study have the same distribution is validated and therefore one can proceed to use the information in the table (see Figure 5.6).

If we focus on the column 'Difference of percentage', the first line indicates the mean effect. Between Cimetidine and Placebo there is a mean difference in efficacy of 23.3% with a 95% confidence interval of 17.2–29.3 (bottom rows). This effect is significant as shown by both the confidence interval (which does not cross 0) and the specific test of statistical significance whose p is reported in the fourth row (0.000).

The other columns show the Odds ratio calculated using the procedures already described. Small differences between results can be noted. They are

	FIXED EFFECT MODEL			
	DIFFERENCE OF PERCENTAGE	LOG ODDS RATIO		
		Peto	Gart	Mantel-Haenszel
Φ	0.233	0.956	0.945	0.982
SE(Φ)	0.031	0.135	0.139	0.140
z	7.547	7.085	6.807	7.014
p(z)	0.000	0.000	0.000	0.000
Q	11.318	8.524	8.617	8.563
p(Q)	0.584	0.808	0.801	0.805
df	13	13	13	13
OR		2.600	2.572	2.671
95%CI	0.293	1.996	1.959	2.030
	0.172	3.387	3.375	3.515

Figure 5.6

due to the difference in the calculations performed for each test, caused in part by the approximation introduced in the method of Gart and Mantel-Haenszel, as described earlier.

Moving from the first to the last row of the table, there is the natural logarithm of the Odds ratio (Φ) for each test, its standard error (SE(Φ)), the significance (z) and its relative p value, the test Q for heterogeneity with its significance (p(Q)) and the degrees of freedom (df) and the Odds ratio (OR) with its confidence interval (95%CI).

ADDITIONAL CONSIDERATIONS ON HETEROGENEITY

In the example shown in Figure 5.6, the test for statistical heterogeneity is not significant and the analysis should be restricted to this section by using the data as presented. However, if the test for statistical heterogeneity is significant, the random effect model must be used.

It is important to note that there is no consensus on how to proceed in the evaluation and interpretation when heterogeneity is present.

If there is statistical heterogeneity, this means that the trials do not belong to the same distribution. A search for the causes of heterogeneity and evaluation of 'outlier trials' needs to be done and analyses with and without outlier trials need to be performed. However, even if the reason for heterogeneity is not detected by a careful review of the trials, the *random effect model* should still be used because it does not have the requirement that all the trials must come from the same distribution. Therefore, the confidence interval is wider and the model is more conservative.

There is a body of opinion that states that the random effect model should always be used, because (a) the results are very similar compared to fixed effect models when statistical heterogeneity is not present, (b) the results from the random models are more 'conservative', and (c) measurements in biology have an intrinsic heterogeneity because of the variability between the individuals. This variability can best be represented by a random effect model.

The author's opinion is that one always needs to remember, as stated by Jenicek, that the purpose of a meta-analysis is not only to calculate a mean effect as a statistical summary, but to derive meaningful evidence for clinical problems that apparently do not have definitive answers.

On this basis, one needs to read the study again in order to understand and interpret information from all the data presented. At the same time, the researcher should be able to form his or her own opinion. This is very important particularly when there is a possible debate on the interpretation of the output, for example, when there is heterogeneity.

The author's suggested algorithm is summarised in Figure 5.7. This suggests that when there is no statistical heterogeneity, one should always use a

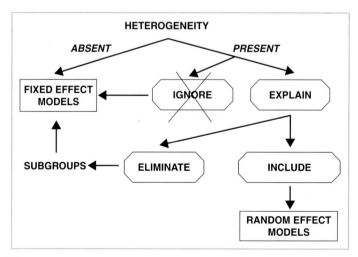

Figure 5.7

fixed effect model. However, for the reasons previously discussed, the result would not change even after using a random effects model. When heterogeneity is present, never ignore it. Read the papers again trying to identify every possible difference in the inclusion criteria, in the exclusion criteria, in the characteristics of the subjects (mean age, co-morbidities, severity of disease) in order to find a way to separate trials into homogeneous groups. If this attempt is successful, the analysis of sub-groups using the fixed effect model will solve the problem. On the other hand, if, by reading the papers, it is found that the statistical heterogeneity is part of the variability of the selected sample of trials and not the effect of differences among the groups of patients or the treatment regimens, then in this case, in this case only, the author recommends for using a random effect model.

The random effects model results can be interpreted using the same criteria as described earlier.

Here the results (Figure 5.8) are very similar to those obtained by the fixed effect model as there is no statistical heterogeneity. If heterogeneity is present, there can be several differences, particularly in the size of the OR confidence interval. The method used to calculate OR in the random effect models is called the DerSimonian–Laird method.

	RANDOM EFFECT MODEL	
	DIFFERENCE OF PERCENTAGE	LOG ODDS RATIO
Φ	0.233	0.945
SE(Φ)	0.031	0.139
z	7.547	6.807
p(z)	0.000	0.000
Q		
p(Q)		
df		
OR		2.572
95%CI	0.293	1.959
	0.172	3.375

Figure 5.8

QUANTIFYING HETEROGENEITY: THE I^2 INDEX

It is known that Cochrane's Q test for heterogeneity has a low statistical power when meta-analyses include few studies. In this case, a cut off value of 10% for significance is more appropriate, even though it is likely to imply higher Type I error (false positive conclusion). Conversely, the test has excessive power to detect clinically unimportant heterogeneity when the meta-analysis includes many studies, particularly mega-trials.

Moreover, this test explores all heterogeneity, not only the true heterogeneity, i.e. the heterogeneity that is due to the actual difference among studies. A very useful approach to this problem is to separate the total variation across studies into the heterogeneity due to true difference (true heterogeneity) and the heterogeneity due to chance. The I^2 index expresses the percentage of the total variation across studies due to heterogeneity. Some authors have arbitrarily indicated the I^2 values of 25%, 50% and 75% as evidence of low, moderate and high heterogeneity, respectively. However, while the I^2 index and its 95% CI are helpful in expressing a quantitative judgment on heterogeneity, these values cannot be considered as categories for decision making.

The program provides the calculation of the I^2 index and its 95% CI for the four methods of calculating Cochrane's Q test.

TESTS FOR PUBLICATION BIAS

The publication bias has already been discussed in the previous chapter.

When the result of a meta-analysis is statistically significant, the publication bias needs to be examined. To do so we can apply three different procedures:

1 *The Publication Bias Assessment according to the Klein formula*: This procedure does not answer the question 'is there or not a publication bias?' but does answer the question: 'if a publication bias is present, how many null or negative studies are needed to void the findings from the meta-analysis?' This data is obtained automatically from the software as an output similar to that shown in Figure 5.9. In this case the test demonstrates that 155 studies with null or negative results are needed to make the meta-analysis show no difference between treatments, and therefore we can consider our results reliable.

There are no guidelines for a practical use of the results of this test. In particular, there is no threshold number that validates the results of meta-analysis. Common sense and practice helps.

PUBLICATION BIAS ASSESSMENT
(number of void or negative trials necessary to render the meta-analysis meaningless.): 116
Number Needed to Treat (95% C.I.): 4 (3/6)
Number Needed to Treat (95% C.I.) (R.E.M.): 4 (3/7)
Test of funnel plot asymmetry: $\alpha=0.45$ 95%C.I.$=-1.36/2.26$ $p(z)=0.63$

Figure 5.9

2 *The Funnel Plot*: A full description of this plot can be found in Chapters 3 and 7.
3 *The test for asymmetry applied on the funnel plot*: Once standardised estimates of ORs (on Y axis) and precision (on X axis) are obtained, for each study a regression line can be drawn. In the absence of publication bias, the intercept on Y axis (α) must be 0. If the 95% CI of α crosses the zero line, we cannot say there is a publication bias. Conversely, if the 95% CI of α does not cross the zero line, we can say there is a publication bias (see also page 53–54). The meta-analysis page shows numerical values of the intercept, its 95% CI, and its *p* value (Figure 5.9).

NUMBER NEEDED TO TREAT (NNT)

Another important and interesting calculation to give a real 'bedside' meaning to the results of meta-analysis is the *Number Needed to Treat (NNT)*. For example, when the aim of a meta-analysis is to evaluate the efficacy of one drug versus another in relation to a one-year survival or to the healing of an ulcer, the NNT indicates how many patients are to be treated to see the one-unit difference between the two treatments. For example, in the evaluation of cimetidine versus placebo in the healing of gastric ulcer, NNT = 4 means that one needs to treat four patients using cimetidine to heal one additional patient compared to Placebo. This information can also be used for some pharmaco-economical evaluations.

When we perform such an evaluation on the efficacy of a new drug, either using a clinical trial or a meta-analysis, the result will lead us to the conclusion whether or not the new drug is significantly more effective than the standard therapy. We will not have the information on the magnitude of the difference between the two strategies (*probabilistic approach*). The NNT measures the effect of a therapy (*quantitative approach*).

This number is calculated as the reverse of the 'pooled risk difference' $\left[\frac{1}{\theta}\right]$, so that two different values are produced depending on the fixed effect model or the random effect model. Both values are calculated by the program, together with their 95% confidence interval (Figure 5.9).

GRAPHICAL REPRESENTATION

The standard plots

In this section, the presentation of results of a meta-analysis using graphical display is illustrated. The figures may be obtained from both fixed effect models and random effect models. In our example, because no heterogeneity was found, the fixed effect model was used to make the graphic plot.

Figure 5.10 shows a standard plot, commonly used and seen in the articles based on meta-analysis. It shows the OR and its confidence interval, represented by a box and two lines on each side of the box, for each individual study. If the confidence interval crosses the vertical line of unity, the result is not statistically significant.

On the left, outside the rectangle, the reference numbers of each trial are shown.

Although all calculations for OR are performed using natural logarithms, OR rather than its logarithm is more appropriate in reporting results as it is easier to interpret. However, the scale needs to be logarithmic so that the two segments of the confidence interval are displayed symmetrically in relation to the central box.

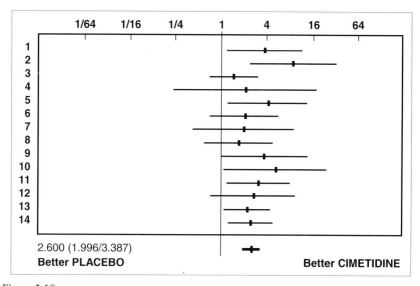

Figure 5.10

All trials show a trend for better efficacy of Cimetidine as compared to Placebo, although some individual trials do not reach statistical significance, in part, due to the small number of patients.

At the bottom, outside the rectangle, the pooled OR shows a statistically significant benefit of Cimetidine.

Although this graph has become the classical way to represent a meta-analysis, it does not give much information. Indeed, it shows only the OR of each study and the pooled OR with their respective confidence interval.

The results may also be expressed as Risk Difference. Figure 5.11 shows this other kind of graph based on the same data set. It is important to note that using the RD, the scale is linear and not logarithmic, and that the line of identity is 0, not 1.

Another graphic plot that gives a more detailed representation of the data is Forest's Plot (Figure 5.12). In this plot, the graphic part is identical to the plots in Figures 5.9 and 5.10, but additional information is added on the side: author, year of publication, number of events/number of subjects included in the study for each group. This kind of graph may also be presented using either the OR-related or the RD-related data.

The plot related to the *cumulative meta-analysis* represents a specific approach to a different problem. An example is shown in Figure 4.12. In this plot, the trials must be listed in a chronological order of publication. The first OR refers to the first trial in time order, the second is the result of a pooled OR between the first and the second trial, the third is the pooled OR

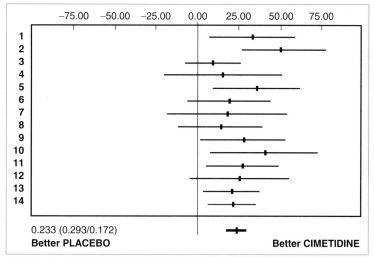

Figure 5.11

46 Chapter 5

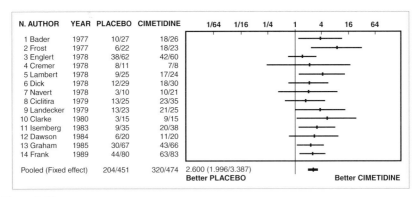

Figure 5.12

among the first three trials, and so on. The last OR is the one resulting from a meta-analysis of all the studies. In other words, this plot shows how every new study added to the previous meta-analysis is able to modify the result of the meta-analysis itself. On the left-hand side of the figure, the number of patients added in every year is listed.

From this graph, one can see that in the year of publication for the first two studies (1977), the results were already definitively in favour of Cimetidine. These results were confirmed in the next year. All subsequent studies after 1978 can be considered as unnecessary or even harmful, because of the risk of adding uncertainty to a problem already solved by the meta-analytical evaluation. These later studies, by adding more patients to the meta-analysis, have allowed a more precise estimation of the OR, which however remains substantially unchanged (the precision is greater when the random error

Figure 5.13

decreases; in this case, the confidence interval becomes smaller, represented by shorter lines).

The cumulative meta-analysis allows a historical evaluation of the data published in the literature and makes possible evaluations unfeasible with the standard meta-analysis. However, the final pooled ORs, whether by the standard or cumulative meta-analysis, are identical.

A similar representation can be obtained by considering the difference of percentage instead of the OR. The way of reading the data is similar, although the scale is not logarithmic in this case and is expressed as a difference of percentage.

The Galbraith plot

The Galbraith plot is a more informative graphical representation. In this graph every trial is represented by a number. The graph axes have two different characteristics: on the x axis the precision of the study (Figure 5.14, line a), as the inverse of the standard error of the OR, or the inverse of the dispersion

$$x = \frac{1}{SE(\Delta)}$$

and on the y axis the standardised OR logarithm (Figure 5.14, line b), which expresses the amount of the effect, given by

$$y = \frac{\Delta}{SE(\Delta)}$$

where $\Delta = \text{Ln OR}$.

Points which are closer to the origin (0,0) indicate poorly informative trials, whereas points far from the origin represent the most precise trials and have more weight in the meta-analysis.

For each trial, one can obtain the OR by drawing a line from the 0,0 point to the logarithmic scale, crossing through the point representing the trial (Figure 5.15, line c). The confidence interval, which is always approximated in a graph, is obtained by drawing two lines between 0,0 and $y \pm 2$ and then reading the value on the scale (Figure 5.15, lines d and e).

The Galbraith plot contains three continuous parallel lines (Figure 5.16, lines f, g and h). The central one, in bold, points to the pooled OR on the scale (line f), the confidence interval is indicated by the segment of arc parallel to the scale (segment i). These three lines, the arc and the numerical values of the OR and of its 95% confidence interval are automatically calculated by the program.

48 Chapter 5

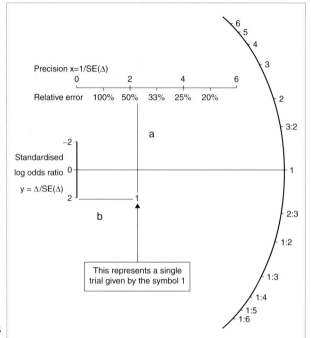

Figure 5.14

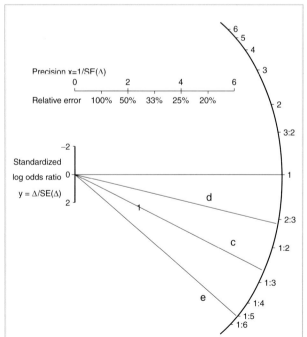

Figure 5.15

Working Procedures   49

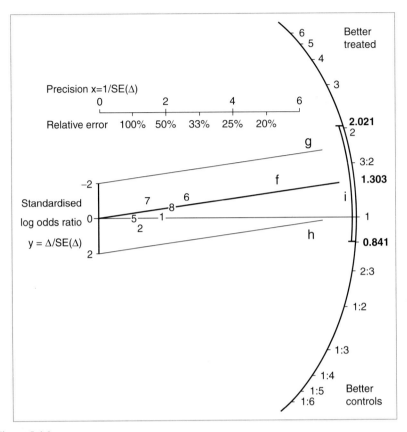

Figure 5.16

The other two lines, originating from 0, ±2 (Figure 5.16, lines g and h), indicate a 'homogeneity area' within their limits. If one or more points (trials) are outside of this area, they are considered as 'heterogeneous'.

If this occurs, we need to undergo all the procedures previously discussed for heterogeneity.

Thus, the Gallbraith plot contains some elements that make it very informative as compared to the traditional plots: it includes the precision (as the inverse of the variance or the dispersion) of every single study, and the homogeneity area identifies which studies are 'outside the mean', establishing heterogeneity in the analysis.

Figure 5.17 shows the Gallbraith plot based on the previously described example of Cimetidine versus Placebo.

One can see that: (1) all the studies are within the homogeneity area; (2) all are in the higher part of the graphic plot; thus, (3) all are in favour of

50 Chapter 5

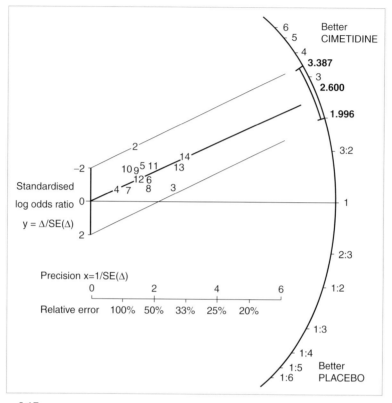

Figure 5.17

Cimetidine; and (4) the relative error (imprecision) is very high in several studies, because these are very small.

Figure 5.18 shows the Gallbraith plot based on the difference in percentage. In this case, the line of equivalence has a value of 0 and the scale, as in the traditional plot, is linear.

The l'Abbè plot

Figure 5.19 shows the l'Abbé plot. In this graphic plot, each trial is again represented by a number. The coordinates on X–Y axes are the proportion of the observed events in the control and treated subjects, respectively.

The solid line represents the points where the event rate in the two groups is identical. The other lines represent the points where a difference of 25% and 50% occurs between the groups.

The size of the circle containing the number of the trial is proportional to the sample size of the trial.

Working Procedures 51

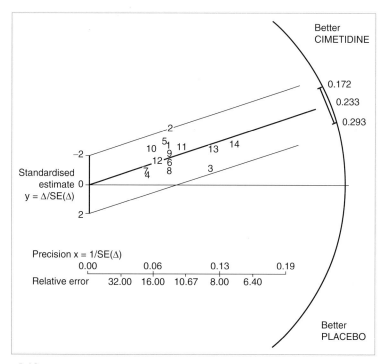

Figure 5.18

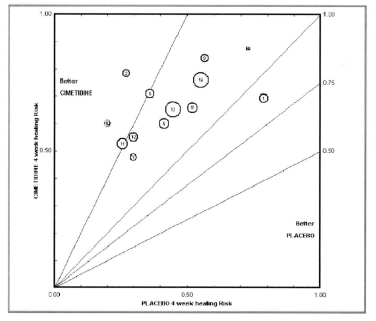

Figure 5.19

52   Chapter 5

This graph can be useful in understanding some of the causes of heterogeneity. Some examples will be discussed later.

The Funnel plot

Figure 5.20 shows an example of the Funnel plot where all the trials are plotted on X–Y axes. The X axis represents the Odds Ratio with a log scale while the Y axis shows the sample size also with a log scale.

The trials included in the Funnel plot seem to be distributed quite symmetrically around the axis represented by the pooled Odds Ratio.

Figure 5.21 shows the plot from a meta-analysis that investigated the effect of a drug aimed at reducing mortality. The Funnel plot shows an obvious asymmetry around the pooled Odds Ratio axis. As shown by the graph, studies with wide sample size are less effective. This may be partly responsible for the asymmetry; however, it may also be due to the absence of published papers with small sample size and negative results.

If using this plot, it should be kept in mind that the results are not quantitative but given by a visual assessment, which may be very obvious in some cases but less so in others.

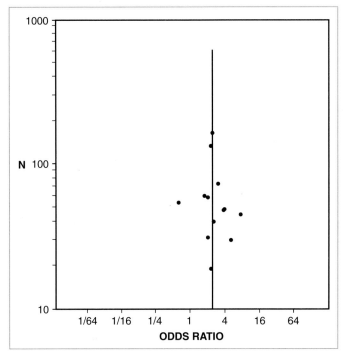

Figure 5.20

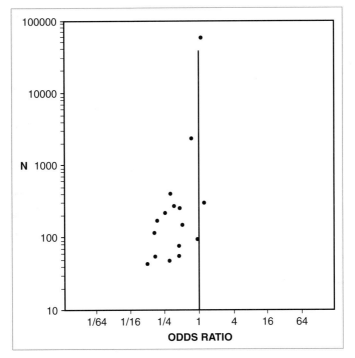

Figure 5.21

The test for asymmetry of the Funnel plot

Figure 5.22 shows the test for asymmetry of the Funnel plot related to cases in Figure 5.20. As shown, 95% CI of the intercept crosses the zero line and therefore indicates there is no significant publication bias.

Figure 5.23 shows the test for asymmetry of the Funnel plot related to cases in Figure 5.21. As shown, 95% CI of the intercept does not cross the zero line and therefore indicates there is a significant publication bias.

The plot for sub-group analysis

Figure 5.24 shows how the sub-group analysis may be helpful to understand a problem in the hetereogeneity of the subjects considered.

A number of studies evaluating the efficacy of Somatostatin in preventing post-ERCP pancreatitis were collected. The meta-analysis, by analysing all the trials, did not show a significant effect of the drug (pooled ORs—represented at the bottom of the figure), but the great variability of efficacy observed in the trials gives rise to the suspicion that something in the trial design or conduct could have caused this difference. Therefore, the trials were divided according to the administration methods of Somatostatin: in

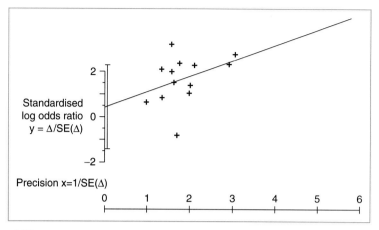

Figure 5.22

three studies, Somatostatin was given by intravenous bolus, in three studies as slow bolus and in five trials by continuous infusion.

The sub-group analysis demonstrates that in the first and third group there is a significant efficacy of the drug, while in the second group no difference was demonstrated compared to Placebo. Whether this is a true reflection of the drug efficacy needs to be assessed with biological clinical trials testing this apparent difference.

This kind of graph, generated by the software program, is easy to read and has the advantage of showing in a single figure, a synthesis of the graphical and numerical results of multiple meta analysis: one for each of the evaluated groups and one for all the groups together. Moreover, both the results of the

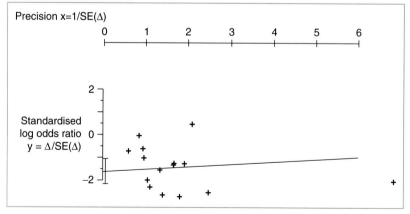

Figure 5.23

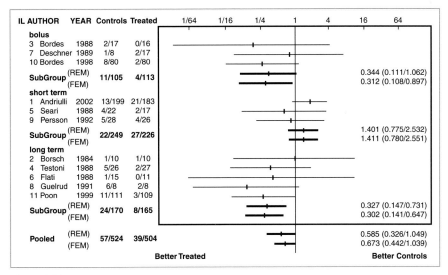

Figure 5.24

pooled ORs, as calculated according to the fixed effect model (FEM) and the random effect model (REM), are displayed.

Using 'flags' while entering the trials in the meta-analysis program allows the trials to be recognised according to their characteristics, which makes the analysis of different sub-groups easy and avoids any modification of the database at this point.

The sub-group analysis is a powerful tool to explore the causes of some differences in the results of the trials that are not dependent on the quality of the drug or the procedure under evaluation.

CHAPTER 6

How to Read, Evaluate and Present a Meta-Analysis

A meta-analysis paper must contain all the details necessary to understand what has been done and how it was done.

By strictly following the rules for the correct execution of a meta-analysis, a good meta-analysis will be obtained. However, in order to give a good interpretation of the results this is not sufficient in itself.

The close collaboration between the meta-analyst and the clinician, an expert in the topic under evaluation, is required in order to accomplish the best interpretation of the results.

HOW TO READ AND EVALUATE A META-ANALYSIS

In reading a scientific paper, one not only tries to learn from other investigators experienced in the subject, but one also evaluates all the procedural and methodological aspects that contribute to the overall value of the work presented. To do so, quality scores have been proposed. They can be applied to evaluate quantitatively and in an objective manner the quality of the article.

In meta-analysis, as in clinical trials, before accepting the conclusions, a critical evaluation has to be performed.

The most commonly used criteria for the evaluation of a meta-analysis are listed in Figure 6.1, which can be easily accessible on-line from: http://york.ac.uk/inst/crd/info.htm

---

Validation of a meta-analysis
The 10 points rule

1. Did the authors work according to a written protocol?
2. Did they carefully describe the questions to be answered by the meta-analysis?
3. Did they clearly describe their research strategy?
4. Did they evaluate the quality of the trials included in the meta-analysis?
5. How was the information summarised?
6. Did they include the characteristics of the patients enrolled in the trials?
7. Did they use a graphic presentation of the results?
8. Did they investigate the outcome heterogeneity?
9. How was the overall therapeutical gain calculated?
10. Was the publication bias taken into account?

Figure 6.1

It is evident that these ten rules comprise all the technical and methodological aspects of a meta-analysis, even though not all authors accept all of them. In particular, Rule 4, while asking whether or not the investigator made sure of the accuracy and scientific value (quality) of the trials included in the analysis, fails to ask how the trials were evaluated. The assessment of the quality of a trial is not part of the final calculations of meta-analysis, but it is essential to gather information for the evaluation of heterogeneity or a sensitivity analysis. Rule 7 asks whether or not the results are reported using a graphic plot, but it does not deal with the accuracy of such a representation. Finally, clinical information on the actual value of the work is not taken into account while evaluating the quality of the meta-analysis. This latter issue represents one of the most important aspects in all the validations and quality assessments.

Figure 6.2 shows our interpretation of the concept of the quality of a meta-analysis, combining methodological concerns with more general considerations on the appropriateness of such an investigation.

> **Validation of a meta-analysis**
> **The golden rules**
>
> 1. Was a RCT the most appropriate way to approach the problem?
> 2. Are sources, inclusion and exclusion criteria, methods and end points clearly defined?
> 3. Did the authors evaluate the homogeneity of the inclusion/exclusion criteria for each trial?
> 4. How were the dropouts evaluated in each trial?
> 5. Was the heterogeneity of the outcome investigated?
> 6. Was the sensitivity evaluated in at least one way?
> 7. Was the publication bias calculated?
> 8. Is the output of the meta-analysis correct and complete?
> 9. Was an expert statistician consulted during the analysis?

Figure 6.2

If an RCT is not the ideal study design for a particular investigation, a meta-analysis should not be performed. Frequently meta-analyses have been performed with RCTs when RCT was not the ideal way to establish the efficacy of a therapy. If such a meta-analysis were to show no evidence of benefit of a particular therapy, then this conclusion would be unsound, firstly because the RCT is not the appropriate study design, and secondly because there may be very few RCTs performed in this particular area.

Another crucial aspect is how to deal with dropouts. They should always be taken into account. Studies that show a 5% dropout should not be included in the same meta-analysis with others that have a 50% dropout rate. These differences may represent important discrepancies between trials. It is a good practice to include studies which have a similar dropout rate, duration of follow-up and so on in a single meta-analysis, and to use sensitivity analyses for trials in which these parameters are very different.

Rule 8 will be addressed below. Rule 9 underlines the importance of a statistician evaluating statistical procedures and a physician interpreting the clinical findings. Therefore, a strong collaboration between these two professionals is essential, in our opinion, to guarantee accuracy and the clinical relevance of a meta-analysis.

HOW TO PRESENT A META-ANALYSIS

There are different ways to present the results of a meta-analysis and the graphic output. This can make it difficult for the reader to evaluate the data correctly and understand how the meta-analysis was carried out. This observation has practical clinical relevance since it is often difficult to decide whether to change one's clinical practice according to the results of a meta-analysis.

When presenting a meta-analysis the data should be provided as numbers (tables) and graphics to help the reader to judge how well the analysis was performed. In particular, we always recommend including:

The number of trials in the meta-analysis
The total number of patients evaluated

This information describes the population studied. It is easy to understand that the relevance and impact of a meta-analysis performed on 50 trials is greater than that of an analysis of three trials. The same consideration applies to the number of subjects studied.

The test for heterogeneity

It is important to know whether the patients included in each single trial have the same distribution. If heterogeneity is present, the investigator should explain how it was interpreted and what has been done to remove it. Heterogeneity can also be represented using graphic plots (the Galbraith plot is preferred over the Funnel plot as the latter has no quantitative evaluation) but it is essential to perform the test and include its result in the paper.

Publication bias assessment (PBA)

PBA is a tool used to assess how many unpublished studies, similar to those published and analysed, are needed to make the results of the meta-analysis not statistically significant. This helps to reinforce the validity of the results provided.

Number needed to treat (NNT)
Odds ratio or risk difference

These data have to be reported numerically as well as using a graphic plot, and each value needs its own confidence interval.

Graphic representation

The standard plot and Forest plot are the most used for graphic representations. The Galbraith plot gives the most complete and informative graphic representation. In fact, it not only shows the effect of the treatment but also the precision and the effect of each single trial included in the meta-analysis. It also provides information on heterogeneity between the trials analysed.

Sub-group analysis

When discrepancies between the size of the effect under evaluation are noted for studies, it is mandatory to look for differences in study design, particularly in the patient inclusion and exclusion criteria, mode of drug administration or dose, or different techniques in surgical or radiological trials.

This will enable the undertaking of an analysis of sub-groups based on these potential differences, which often allow a better understanding of the data, for example assessing the direct relationship between the efficacy of treatment and some specific characteristic of trial design, including characteristics of patients, e.g. old versus young.

EXAMPLES

A few examples of correct representations of a meta-analysis are shown below.

In the first example (Figure 6.3) the upper left corner shows the subject of the meta-analysis, trials of Interferon versus placebo for the treatment of hepatitis C. The meta-analysis was performed with the selection of 15 trials including a total number of 767 patients (upper right corner). The Galbraith plot shows that all the trials were similar for individual precision of the estimate of the effect, and there was no heterogeneity.

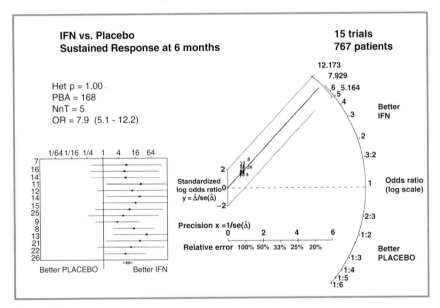

Figure 6.3

From this graphic representation it is possible to conclude that Interferon is an effective drug. The PBA is 168, indicating that the analysis is very reliable. NNT and Odds ratio are also represented together with their confidence intervals.

The second example (Figure 6.4) shows the sustained anti-viral response, following 6 months Interferon alone versus Interferon + Ribavirin for the

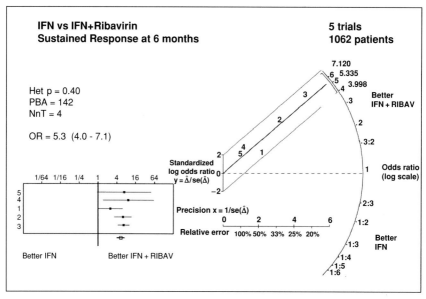

Figure 6.4

treatment of hepatitis C. Five trials were included in the analysis and the total number of patients was 1062.

The Galbraith plot clearly shows that two out of the five trials have a precision significantly higher than that of the other three, indicating that these two studies can be considered as 'mega-trials' (i.e. a greater number of patients were included).

This way of illustrating the results of a meta-analysis is the most complete and accurate for any software.

CHAPTER 7

How to Use the Program

The program is easy and intuitive to use as it is a Windows-based program.

The handbook will describe in detail all the functions of the program; possible problems are explored.

GENERAL INFORMATION

META is a program for META-ANALYSIS. It has a database into which it is easy to enter the original data and to elaborate the data statistically. The graphic section allows a visual representation of this data and allows it to be printed using any Windows-supported printer.

Although one can use this program without specific training, this part of the handbook provides useful information in order to use it properly to its full potential.

Minimum requirement of the system
Processor: PENTIUM III (or compatible);
Operative system: Windows 9x/ME/XP/2000.
Memory: 64 MB of conventional memory free;
Hard disk with at least 10 MB free;
Colour Monitor with a resolution of at least 800 × 600;
Printer any Laserjet or InkJet Windows-supported.

Main characteristics of the program
The program is designed to
- save a large number of studies organised in one or more databases and to easily modify data already entered;
- create and save data regarding multiple endpoints for each individual study with an easy and fast evaluation these data;
- select only a part of the data entered for a separate evaluation;
- sort the inserted studies for different fields, with a simple click of the mouse;
- produce an analytical or graphic output (derived from results of the calculations) for the video or for the printer. The program is compatible with most printers, and it generates printouts with high resolution graphics;
- select the format of the output according to individual needs, avoiding the printing of unnecessary results.

The program is entirely written in Delphi language and it uses archives in Paradox format.

INSTALLATION OF THE PROGRAM

To install the program on a computer follow these steps:
1 Insert the installation CD (auto-starting), then wait for the automatic start of the installation program.

2 If the installation program does not start automatically, click on the icon 'My computer' on the screen, then on the CD drive and double-click on the Setup.exe icon.
3 Follow the instructions of the installation program (all the CD files will be transferred to the hard disk).

STRUCTURE OF THE PROGRAM

The program 'Metanalysis' has been designed to work with all operative systems that are Windows-based. Thus, the characteristic of its structure is similar to all standard Windows programs.

Main features of the program
The program window will open in this way:

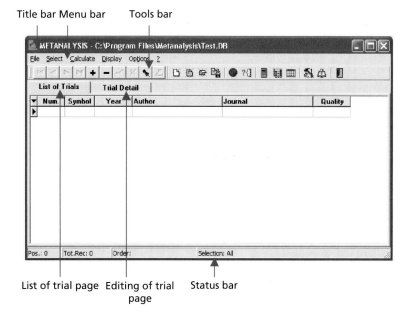

Title bar
Shows the program title 'Metanalysis', followed by the complete path name of the current trial.

Menu bar
It contains the menu items for different program functions.

Some of the menu items have a sub-menu that can be seen by clicking the item selected.
To open the selected function, click over the item.
A short description of the different functions of the menu is given below (the symbol '/' indicates the separation between the main menu item and the sub-menu item).

File/New
To create a new archive file.

File/Open
To open an existing archive file. The program, when started, automatically opens the last meta-analysis used by the program. Therefore, one needs to use this function only when moving from one meta-analysis to another.

File/Save as...
To save the meta-analysis on a file different from that in use, or on a floppy disk or another drive, or to transfer the meta-analysis to another computer.

Close
To close the meta-analysis.

Exit from Metanalysis
To exit completely from the program.

Select/All trials
To see all the meta-analysis trials without any selection filter.

Select/Simple select
To add a selection filter to the meta-analysis trials using the most significant fields. Only the selected trials will be shown and the calculation will be done on them.

Select/Advanced select
Another function to add some selection filters. It differs from the previous one since it utilizes all the fields. It can be used especially by those familiar with the SQL language (*System Query Language*).

Select/Display/Execute SQL query
To show and modify the SQL query relative to the current selection. Useful only for those who are familiar with the SQL language.

Calculate
To calculate the meta-analysis using only the selected trials. This computation is necessary to obtain the output both in text format and in graphic form.

Display/Graphic Results
After having used the function 'calculate', it is possible with this function to see and print the results of the final calculations in a graphic format. Different types of graphs are available and will be described in later sections.

Display/Analytic Results
To see and print the results of the calculation in text format.

Display/Variables
To see the values of the main variables used by the program. It is useful if a debugger program needs to be used.

Options
To set different options of the program.

Tools bar
It contains a series of buttons to rapidly access the main functions of the program.
The first series of buttons are grouped in a tools bar that allows display and editing of different trials.
The other buttons are similar to those used for the other menu items.
The buttons are not always active. When a program function is not available, the corresponding button is not activated and appears in grey.
When moving the mouse pointer over a button, the program will show a message explaining the button function for a few seconds.

Status bar
Shows the following information:
- the position of the trial inside the table;
- the total number of selected trials;
- the order of the included trials;
- the page of the list of trials;
- a global view in a grid form of the trials included in the table;
The user has the opportunity to select part of the trials and only these will be seen in the grid.

The grid shows only the most significant data of the trials; to have a complete list of the trials one needs to go to the 'Trial Detail' page.

Trial Detail page

This page shows in detail the data of each single trial and allows editing of every part of its data.

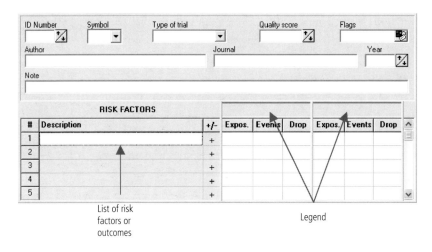

ID number
A numeric field to identify a trial in a unique way. It can be shown, instead of the 'Symbol' field, to identify the trial in the different graphical and analytical outputs.

Symbol
This field also identifies a trial in a unique way. It can be used instead of the field 'ID Number'.

Type of trial
It can be either a 'Full paper' or an 'Abstract'. To select one of the two options just click over the text cell.

Quality score
It can be a number included between 0 and 100. It can be useful to order the trials in different outputs.

Flags
This field allows the attachment of 'flags' to indicate with characters (up to 10) some characteristics of the study. It is possible to use any kind of character; every character will identify a characteristic. Later, during analysis, it will be possible to select all studies having a specific characteristic. For

example: 'MC' might have the meaning of 'Male Children'. When a new flag is added (never used before during the meta-analysis), it is necessary to edit the table of flags by clicking over the button next to the text cell and adding it to the specific table of the new flag and its description.

Author
Name of the first author who published the article.

Journal
Name of the journal, in full or abbreviated form.

Year
Year of publication of the study.

Note
Any note up to a maximum of 100 characters.

RISK FACTORS description
It is possible to add more than one 'Risk Factor' (survival, side effects, length of stay, etc.). In the phase of computation it will be possible to choose any particular risk factor for evaluation using the meta-analysis.

+/−
The character '+' or '−' indicates if the event under study is a positive event (recovery, survival, etc.) or a negative one (recurrence, death, etc.). This will modify the insertion of some legends in the figures.

Exposed–Events–Drop
The numeric values to be inserted for every trial and every factor. In the heading of these columns the corresponding legend should be indicated.

File format
For each meta-analysis the program generates two files on the disk: one with the ".DB" extension, which is a database table in paradox format; the other has the '.INI' extension, which is a configuration file. The name and the allocation of these two files are decided by the user.

USE OF THE PROGRAM

This chapter does not contain any information regarding the Windows operating system. For any problem concerning this topic we recommend referring to a Windows user manual.

GETTING STARTED

To start the program, double-click the Metanalysis icon on the desktop. If you do not find the Metanalysis icon on the desktop, try clicking over the START menu Programs\Metanalysis.

When you open the program for the first time, you will see the following window:

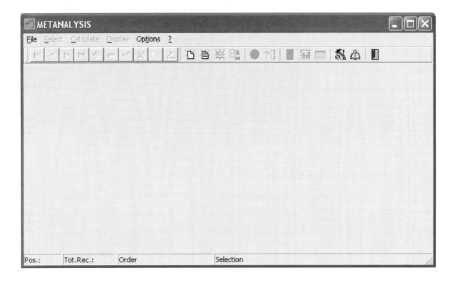

It is now necessary to create a new file, as explained in detail in the following section.

How to create a new metanalysis file
Select from the menu the field File/New or click over the tools bar button.
A dialogue box will appear to choose the name of the file.
Write the name for the new file inside the text cell 'File name' i.e. 'Test' (the file's name should respect the file's name rules for Windows).
Confirm by clicking over the 'Open' button.
   The following program window will appear:

To add a new trial
Click **+** over the tools bar button. If the page currently in use is the 'List of trials' page, the edit page 'Trial Detail' will appear automatically and it will be possible to add the trial's data.

How to Use the Program 71

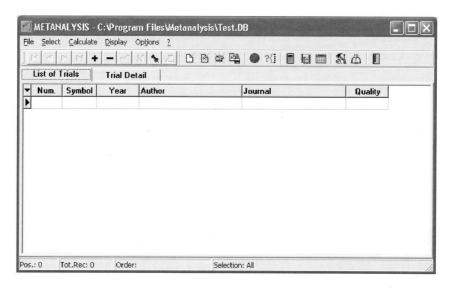

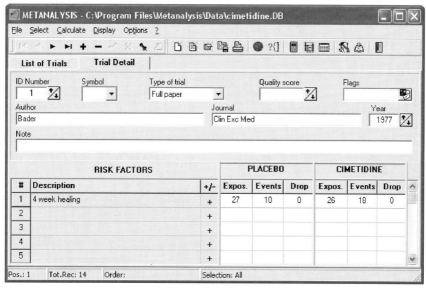

To confirm the inserted data in this page and save them, you need to click ✓ over the tools bar button; to delete them click over the button ✗.

To modify a pre-existing trial

If the page currently in use is the 'List of trials', you need to first open the 'Trial detail' page by clicking over the specific icon or double-clicking the grid row. It is now possible to modify any field of the trial.

Be aware that the fields with grey background (Description, +/− and the two legends) are global and if you make a change to these data, the change will affect all the trials in the meta-analysis file.

How to save the meta-analysis

Usually, you do not need to save the meta-analysis file, because the program will automatically save the file while you are working on or updating the file.

However, you may want to save the meta-analysis file with a different name, in a different folder of the hard-disk or in another drive to move it to another computer. In these cases, select from the menu the item 'File/Save as...'.

A new dialogue window will appear where you will indicate the new folder or the new file name. The file name must have the '.DB' extension that will automatically be added by the program.

The saved meta-analysis will be the active one on the program.

How to select the trials for analysis

Usually, the program works on all the trials included in the table for the meta-analysis.

However, one can decide to select only a part of the trials for the meta-analysis.

To easily set some selection criteria for the trials, click over the menu item 'Select/Simple select' or over the toolbar button.

The program will now show the windows with a form to define the selection criteria.

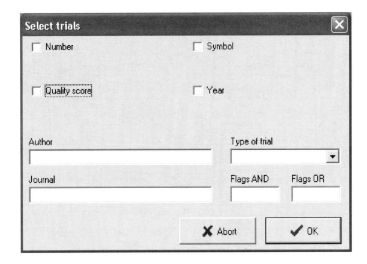

Add to the form ONLY the data necessary for the selection.

For example, if selecting all the trials with an ID number greater than or equal to 10, published in the 1980s and not including the abstracts, you should fill in the form like this:

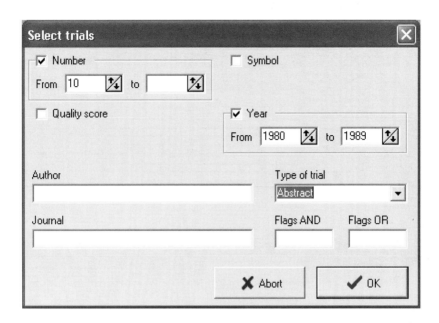

More details are needed for the two selection fields 'Flags AND' and 'Flags OR'; these fields allow selection based on the 'flags' added to the different trials.

In each field you can insert multiple characters, each one related to a flag.

The characters inserted in the 'Flags AND' field must be present in the Flags field of the trials to be selected; on the other hand, by adding more than one character in the 'Flags OR' field, the program will select all the trials in which at least one of the inserted characters is present in the Flags field.

For example, let us assume that in the table trial we have four trials with the following flags: trial 1 'BCM', trial 2 'AB', trial 3 'CDE', trial 4 'M'.

If in the 'Flags AND' field we write the character 'BM', only the first trial will be selected, because it is the only one containing both the flag 'B' and 'M'.

If in the 'Flags OR' field we write the characters 'BM', three trials will be selected: the first, the second and the fourth, because in these three trials at least one character contained in this field is present.

Advanced Select

This function, like the previous one, permits selection of the trials to be evaluated, but it works in a different way and it is reserved for those who are familiar with the internal structure of the trial table and are familiar with SQL (System Query Language).

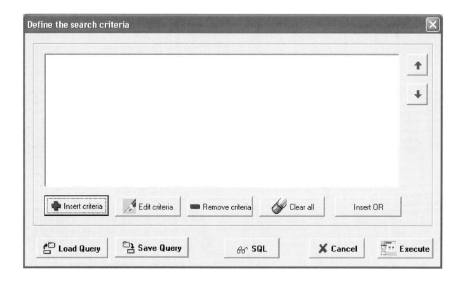

The **Insert criteria** button allows insertion of a new selection criterion. A window will appear where it will be possible to select the field for the selection, the operator and the value to be compared.

For example, if one wants to select all the trials with an ID Number > 4, one needs to fill the window as follows:

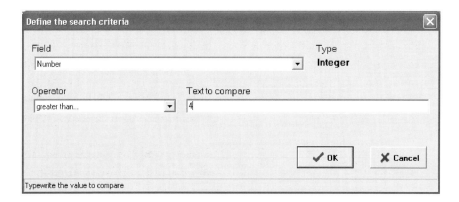

It is possible to insert multiple selection criteria. Each criterion has its own row in the space of the window.

With the buttons ↑ and ↓ you can invert the row order.

Each row contains a single variable or characteristic. The program automatically defaults to associating these together by the operation AND. To change this selection the operator AND is changed to OR by clicking the button **Insert OR**.

If you want to select all the trials with an ID Number > 4 or the 'B' character in the Flags field, the selection window will appear as follows:

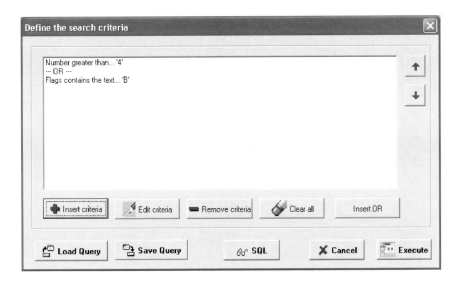

To modify a criterion, double click over the specific row or click over the **Edit criteria** button, after having selected the row with the mouse.

To delete a criterion, use the **Remove criteria** button.

To delete all the selection criteria, click the **Clear all** button.

After having set the different selection criteria, the **Save Query** and **Load Query** buttons will save all the selection criteria inserted, which will be saved on the file for later operations.

The **Execute** button will generate and perform the SQL instruction related to the inserted criteria. As a result, in the trials table only the selected trials will appear.

The **SQL** button shows the SQL instruction generated by the program. Those familiar with SQL may modify the instruction according to their needs.

76 Chapter 7

How to show all the trials
After having selected the trials, having removed the selection filter in order to show all the trials included in the meta-analysis file, select the **Select/All trials** function or click ● over the tools bar button.

Calculate
This is the function that performs the analysis on the selected trials and calculates all the meta-analysis data. During this phase, it is possible to send the output of the calculation directly to the printer. In every case, the results are saved for further outputs either to the screen or printer.

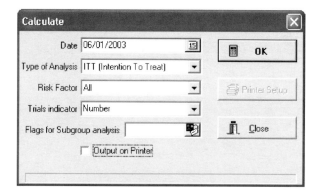

All the form fields must be filled before starting the calculation.

The **Date** is the date of calculation and it will appear on the outputs. One can modify it by typing or by clicking the button on the right-hand side of the text cell using the mouse.

The **Type of Analysis** field may be 'ITT (Intention To Treat)' or 'PP (Per Protocol)'. By selecting one of these procedures, the meta-analysis will be performed according to the calculation described in Chapter 5.

Risk Factor may be either 'All' or only one of the Risk factors inserted in the meta-analysis table. By selecting one of the risk factors, the program will perform the calculation considering only that factor. If one selects 'All' instead, the program subsequently elaborates all the Risk factors. In this case it is necessary to check the **Output on Printer** field in order to obtain the output on the printer, because only the data from the last Risk factor is automatically fully saved and available for the output.

The **Trial indicator** field may be 'Number', 'Symbol' or 'Point'. These are three different ways to identify each trial in the graphic or numerical outputs.

The **Flags for Sub-group analysis** field allows a 'Sub-group analysis' output. In practice, if one inserts a number of flags in this field (used for the different trials), it is possible to obtain a graphic output with the data of the trials grouped according to these flags.

The **OK** button starts the calculation process that will last a variable period of time depending on the number of trials selected and the computer's performance.

If the check box **Output on Printer** is checked, the printed output will occur at the same time with the calculation. In any case, the data of the last elaborated risk factor will be saved automatically.

Graphic Results

Once the meta-analysis has been completed, it can be shown on the screen or printed on paper in different graphic formats. To activate this function, select the item '**Display/Graphic result**' from the menu or click over the tools bar button.

The following window will produce an output either on screen or printer by selecting the specific page (click either one of the icons on the upper part of the window).

Output on Screen

Just select one of the different **plot types**, the **Model** and the **Pooled result**, then click the **Display** button.

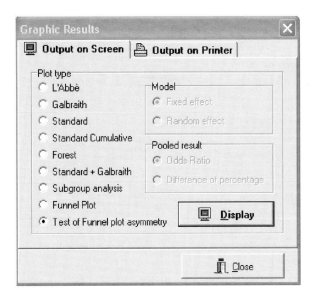

Chapter 7

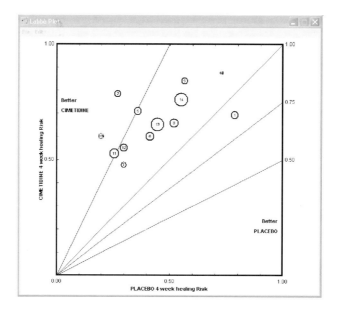

Example of the L'Abbè plot.

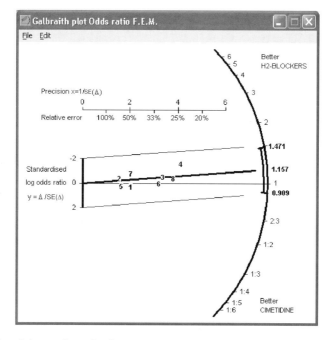

Example of the Galbraith plot.

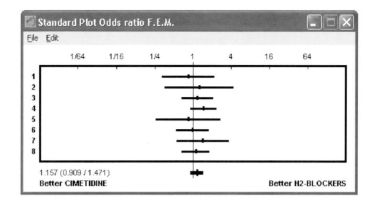

Example of a Standard plot.

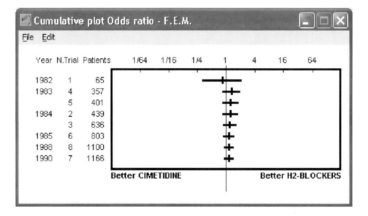

Example of a Standard cumulative plot.

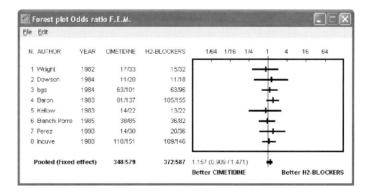

Example of the Forest plot.

When this graph is shown on screen:

It is possible to **set the size** of the graph by clicking over the windows borders and moving the mouse in the direction desired without releasing the mouse button.

With the **File/Save to** item you can save the graphic plot on file (BMP format).

File/Print prints the graph on paper (it is better to use the specific print function for the graphs described below).

Edit/Copy to clipboard uses the Windows clipboard to copy the graph image and then paste it over in any Windows program that utilizes the clipboard, such as PowerPoint or Word.

Output on Printer

By selecting this page you can send the graphic output to the printer.

Different printing modalities may be selected for the graphics, which will be sent to an A4 format paper.

The program will arrange different graphs over a sheet of paper.

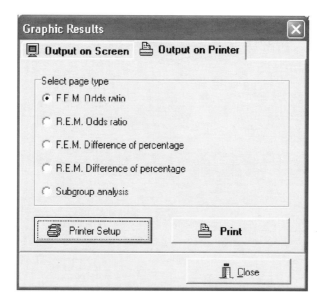

The **Printer Setup** button allows one to choose the printer to use and the modalities of printing.

The **Print** button starts the printing.

How to Use the Program

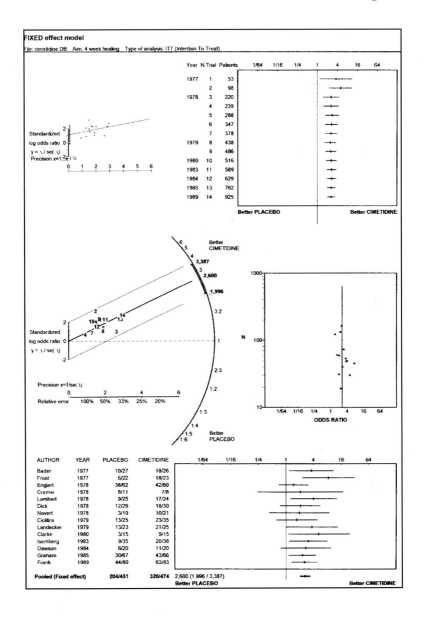

Examples of printing of an F.E.M. Odds ratio.

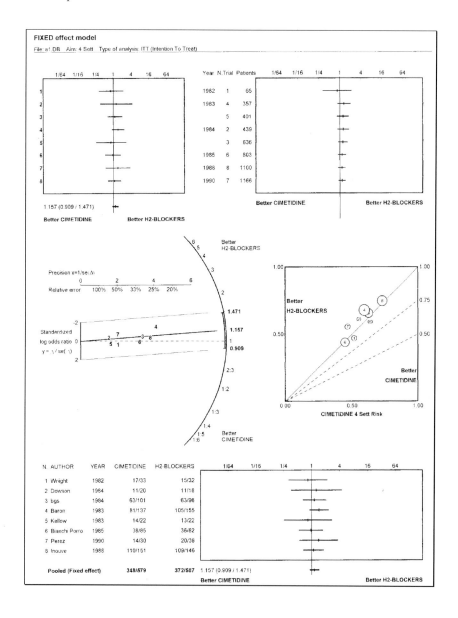

Analytical Result

You can show and print the data of the meta-analysis in a numerical format.

This function will be activated by selecting the item **Display/Analytical result** from the menu or by clicking 🏛 on the tools bar button.

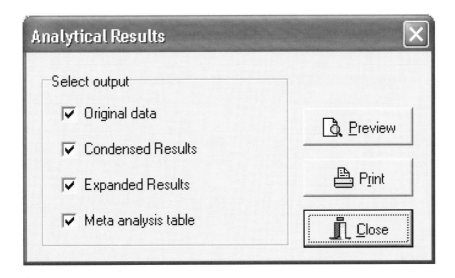

In this window you can choose different output formats that you want. The **Print** button will directly execute the printing of the data.

The **Preview** button will show the data on the screen as they will be printed.

File: a1.DB - Aim: 4 Sett
Type of analysis: ITT (Intention To Treat)
Date: 26/01/2003

ORIGINAL DATA							
Author	Journal	Score	Year	CIMETIDINE		H2-BLOCKERS	
				Ent.	Obs.	Ent.	Obs.
1 Wriight	Mpf	22	1982	33	17	32	15
2 Dowson	Scand	0	1984	20	11	18	11
3 bgs	gUT	0	1984	101	63	96	63
4 Baron	Scand	0	1983	137	81	155	105
5 Kellow	Digestion	0	1983	22	14	22	13
6 Bianchi Porro	Digestion	0	1985	85	38	82	36
7 Perez	Curr	2	1990	30	14	36	20
8 Inouve	Drugs	94	1988	151	110	146	109
			TOTALS	579	348	587	372

Example of Original Data.

Chapter 7

File: cimetidine.DB - Aim: 4 week healing
Type of analysis: ITT (Intention To Treat)
Date: 28/01/2004

METANALYSIS

	FIXED EFFECT MODEL				RANDOM EFFECT MODEL	
	DIFFERENCE OF PERCENTAGE	LOG ODDS RATIO			DIFFERENCE OF PERCENTAGE	LOG ODDS RATIO
		Peto	Gart	Mantel Haenszel		
Φ	0,233	0,956	0,945	0,982	0,233	0,945
SE(Φ)	0,031	0,135	0,139	0,140	0,031	0,139
z	7,547	7,085	6,807	7,014	7,547	6,807
p(z)	0,000	0,000	0,000	0,000	0,000	0,000
Q	11,318	8,524	8,617	8,563		
p(Q)	0,584	0,808	0,801	0,805		
df	13	13	13	13		

I² is the percentage of total variation across studies due to heterogeneity rather than chance

I²	0,0	0,0	0,0	0,0		
95%CI	52,3 / 0,0	36,7 / 0,0	37,4 / 0,0	37,0 / 0,0		

OR		2,600	2,572	2,671		2,572
95%CI	0,293 / 0,172	1,996 / 3,387	1,959 / 3,375	2,030 / 3,515	0,293 / 0,172	1,959 / 3,375

Quality Adjusted

QA	0,233		2,572			
95%CI	0,172 / 0,293		1,959 / 3,375			

PUBLICATION BIAS ASSESSMENT
(number of void or negative trials necessary to render the meta-analysis meaningless.): 155

Number Needed to Treat (95% C.I.): 4 (3 / 6)
Number Needed to Treat (95% C.I.) (R.E.M.): 4 (3 / 6)
Test of funnel plot asymmetry: α = 1,15   95%C.I.= -0,16 / 2,47   p(z)=0,09

Example of a Meta-analysis Table page.

Options

This function allows the setting of some parameters of the program.
The different set-ups are divided into three sections:

Fonts

You can choose the type of font that the program should use while showing the graphs and the symbols identifying the trials.

How to Use the Program 85

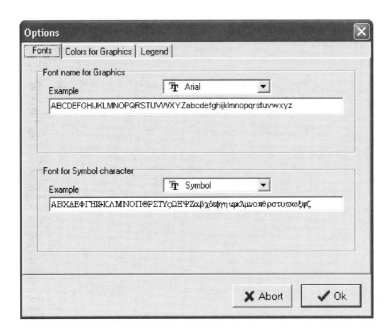

Colours for Graphics

In this section you can choose the colour for the background, the lines and the data on the graphs.

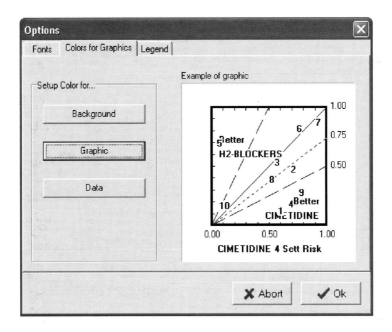

86   Chapter 7

By clicking over one of the three buttons a window will be opened for the choice of colour.

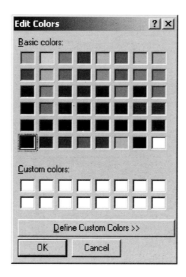

Legend

To set a legend that will be shown on the graphs.

You can choose between two fixed items ('Better' and 'Favour') or indicate a personalised item.

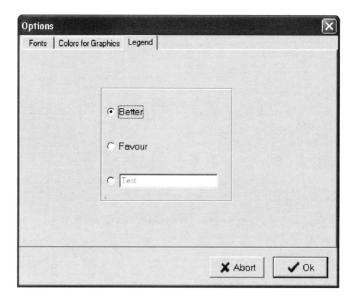

References

C.D. Mulrow. Rationale for systematic reviews. *BMJ* 309: 597–599, 1994.

K. Pearson Report on certain enteric fever inoculation statistics. *BMJ* 3:1243–1246, 1904.

R.A. Fisher. *Statistical Methods for Research Workers*. London: Oliver and Boyd, 1932.

A. Whitehead, N.M.B. Jones. A Meta-analysis of clinical trials involving different classifications of response into ordered categories. *Stat Med* 13: 2503–2515, 1994.

V. Hasselblad, D.C. McCrory. Meta-analytic tools for medical decision making: a practical guide. *Med Decis Making* 15: 81–96, 1995.

S.G. Thompson. Why sources of heterogeneity in meta-analysis should be investigated. *BMJ* 309: 1351–1355, 1994.

A. Whitehead, J. Whitehead. A general paramentric approach to the meta-analysis of randomized clinical trials. *Stat Med* 10: 1665–1677, 1991.

S. Klein, J. Simes, G.L. Blackburn. Total parenteral nutrition and cancer clinical trial. *Cancer* 58: 1378–1386, 1986.

T.C. Chalmers. Problems induced by meta-analysis. *Stat Med* 10: 971–980, 1991.

K.A. L'Abbè, A.S. Detsky, K. O'Rourke. Meta-analysis in clinical research. *Ann Int Med* 107: 224–233, 1987.

R.F. Galbraith. A note on graphical presentation of estimated odds ratios from several clinical trials. *Stat Med* 7: 889–894, 1988.

D.T. Felson. Bias in meta-analytic research. *J Clin Epidemiol* 45: 885–892, 1992.

D. Petitti. *Meta-analysis, Decision Analysis and Cost-effectiveness Analysis (Methods for quantitative synthesis in medicine)*, Oxford: Oxford University Press.

H. Cooper, L.V. Hedges eds. *Handbook of Research Synthesis*. New York: Russel Sage Foundation, 1994.

JPT Higgins, SG Thompson. Quantifying heterogeneity in a meta-analysis. *Stat Med* 21: 1539–1558, 2002.

GLOSSARY

Bias. Introduction of a systematic error in a procedure that leads to a wrong estimate of a phenomenon. In a meta-analysis there are several potential biases that need to be controlled. The most important is the 'publication bias'.

Capture–mark–recapture method. Method used for estimating data that could not be measured by traditional assessment methods.

Cumulative meta-analysis plot. Approach that shows how much any new study added to the previous meta-analysis is able to modify its result.

Evidence-based medicine. Approach to clinical problems aimed at the integration of individual clinical expertise with the best clinical evidence available from a systematic review. In other words EBM is the use of both evidence and experience in clinical practice.

Fixed and random effects models. Calculations performed under two different hypotheses. In the first hypothesis, the effects evaluated are expected to be part of the same distribution. If this assumption is not met, it means that the studies are sampled from a population that includes several different populations, each provided with its own mean. In this case, it could be necessary to use a random effect model.

Grey literature. It is the name given to material produced by government, academies, business and industries; both in print and electronic formats, but which is not controlled by commercial publishing interests and where publishing is not the primary activity of the organisation.

Heterogeneity. In meta-analysis, it refers to the various responses to a given treatment among the included studies. It might relate to the biological difference among the individuals, but also to other differences that are not always detectable. The statistical heterogeneity may be assessed through specific tests (test for heterogeneity) and also the extent to which the heterogeneity is due to chance may be evaluated (I^2 Index).

Intention-to-treat (ITT) analysis. Strategy of analysis in which all randomised patients are analysed, even though they have not completed the treatment. They are considered cases of therapeutic failure.

Meta-analysis. Method that aims to reach the comprehensive synthesis of data issued from a systematic research and to analyse congruent and divergent findings from reports in literature. It should be the methodological ground of a systematic review.

Number needed to treat (NnT). It is the number of patients that one needs to treat with the drug under study to heal one patient more than placebo or reference drug. It is a 'bed-side' measure of therapeutic gain. It is easy to calculate:

$$NnT = \frac{1}{RD} \text{ or } \frac{1}{\text{pooled RD}}.$$

It is an integer number and its approximation is to the higher integer.

Outcomes. All that can be the subject of a clinical study. If we are investigating the effect of a drug on recovery from a certain disease, outcomes might be the recovery itself, side effects, mortality, data related to the drug administration, etc.

Per-protocol (PP) analysis. Strategy of analysis in which only patients who completed the trial are analysed. It is useful when we are interested in knowing the real efficacy of a drug.

Plot. Graph in which two quantities or a quantity and a group of categories are put in relationship. The most used plots in meta-analysis are those of Forrest, Galbraith, L'Abbè, the Funnel plot and the cumulative meta-analysis plot.

Quality score. Rating the quality of the studies which are to be included in the meta-analysis, verifying the presence in them of some 'markers of quality' defined before starting the evaluation procedure. It is useful for sensitivity analyses.

Randomised controlled trial (RCT). This is a clinical study with two major characteristics: randomisation and the presence of a control group.

Risk. In an epidemiological/statistical context, it is the proportion of an event (death, healing and success of a therapy). In other words, the number of events divided by the number of studied cases. If we observe 320 cases of gastric ulcer healing in 474 patients treated with cimetidine, the proportion or the risk of healing is 67.5%.

$$\frac{320}{474} = 0.675.$$

It should be remarked that within this context the term 'risk' does not involve a negative judgment on the observed event, even though the negative events are called 'risk', and positive events called 'benefit increase'.

The **95% Confidence Interval (CI)** is used to study the inconsistency of the estimate of a risk. It is the interval of the estimate obtained if the study is replicated n times on 800 subjects.

The interval is calculated according to the following formula:

$$p \pm 1.96 * SE(p)$$

where p is the proportion (which is 0.675 in our example) and $SE(p)$ is the standard error of p.

$$SE(p) = \sqrt{p * (1 - p)/n}$$

where n is the total number of the subjects of the study. Continuing with our example of ulcer healing,

$$0.675 \pm 1.96\sqrt{0.675 * 0.325/474}$$

$$0.675 \pm 0.042$$

$$95\% CI = 0.633 - 0.717.$$

If we are studying another population of subjects with gastric ulcer treated with placebo and observing 204 healings out of 451 subjects, the following table can be used:

	Healing		Total
	Yes	No	
Cimetidine	320	154	474
Placebo	204	247	451

We can thus calculate the following:

Risk difference (RD)

$$\frac{320}{474} - \frac{204}{451} = 0.675 - 0.452 = 0.223$$

The difference of the proportion of the events observed in the two groups refers to the therapeutic gain (+22.3%). In epidemiological terms the RD is known as **Absolute Risk Reduction (ARR)**.

Risk ratio (RR)

$$\frac{320}{474} \bigg/ \frac{204}{451} = 1.49.$$

It refers to the extent to which the frequency of an event (in our example, the recovery from gastric ulcer) can vary in the presence of the factor we are studying (treatment with cimetidine) compared to absence of the latter (placebo).

Odds ratio (OR). A measure that is similar to the Risk Ratio because it refers to the estimate of the latter when the event is not frequent ($\leq 10\%$). It is calculated as follows:

$$\frac{320 * 247}{154 * 204} = \frac{79040}{31416} = 2.52.$$

If the Risk Difference or the Odds Ratio is calculated from a meta-analysis, and therefore from more studies, they are called **pooled RD** or **pooled OR**.

Systematic research. Complete literature search throughout all potential data sources by means of defined procedures aiming at the inclusion of all aspects of the search question.

Systematic review. Review performed by an expert in the field based not only on the knowledge of the single investigator but also on data issued from a systematic research.

Index

absolute risk reduction 13, 25, 92
abstract
   bibliographic search for 10
   inclusion and exclusion for meta-analysis 10
   for scientific paper reading 10
Advanced Select option of META program
   Clear all button 75
   Edit criteria button 75
   Execute button 75
   Insert criteria button 74
   Insert OR button 75
   Load Query button 75
   Remove criteria button 75
   Save Query button 75
   SQL button 75
analytical results display in META program 82. *See also* graphic results display in META program
ARR. *See* absolute risk reduction
articles
   evaluating 10
   finding 10
   reading 11

bias
   extractor 19
   follow-up time 20
   geographical 19
   inclusion criteria 18
   indexing 18
   introduction in scoring systems 12
   meta-analyst caused 19
   in meta-analytical research 15
   multiple publication 18
   multiple used subjects 18
   publication 9, 16, 18
   quality score 19
   recording error 19
   reference 18
   reporting 19
   search 18
   selector 18
bibliographic search for abstracts 10
bibliographic sources 8. *See also* medical bibliographic sources
biomedical interest
   grey literature 9
   use of meta-analysis 4

capture–mark–recapture method 89, 20
Chapman method 21
check list for scientific paper reading 10
chi-square
   distribution 5, 25, 29
   for heterogeneity 30
CI. *See* confidence interval
Cimetidine versus Placebo trials
   data accuracy example 34
   Galbraith plot 47, 49
   l'Abbè plot 51
   number needed to treat 43
   standard plot 44, 45, 46
   trials output evaluation 36, 37
clinical research objectives 5
clinical trials 58
   characteristics choosing 8
Cochrane's Q test for homogeneity 42
β-coefficient calculation 31
collection of published literature 3
confidence interval 21
   95% confidence interval 91
   in fixed effects models 26
confidence interval estimation
   by Mantel-Haenszel method 27
   by Peto method 29
   for trials output evaluation 36, 37

conformity publication bias 16
cumulative meta-analysis 14, 45
  plot 89

data accuracy
  Cimetidine drug effect example 34
  intention to treat analysis 35
  per protocol analysis 35
  Placebo drug effect example 34
data collection for meta-analysis
  design of trial information 12
  flags 13
  generic information 11
  outcomes 12
  quality score 12
  study and control group treatment 12
data reliability 9
degrees of freedom 5, 25, 29
DerSimonian–Laird method 30, 41
difference of percentage
  calculation 25
  estimation for trials output evaluation 36
  in fixed effect model 38, 39
dispersion 24, 47

Embase 8
evidence-based medicine 89
extractor bias 19

FEM. See fixed effects models
file format in META program 69
Fisher's inverse chi-squared method 5
fixed effects models 13, 24, 89
  difference of percentage calculation 25
  Gart estimations 39
  Mantel-Haenszel method 26, 39
  Peto method 28, 39
  pooled effect evaluation 38
  statistical heterogeneity and 40
  sub-group analysis 55
  test for heterogeneity 25
  See also random effects models
flags information 13
follow-up time bias 20
Fonts function in META program 84
Funnel plot
  method 16
  odds ratio calculation 52, 53
  for publication bias assessment 43
  test for asymmetry 43, 53
  See also Galbraith plot; l'Abbè plot

Galbraith plot 47
  Cimetidine versus Placebo trials 50
  log odds ratio estimation 48

precision estimation 48
  See also Funnel plot; l'Abbè plot
gastric ulcer (data accuracy example) 34
generic information 11
geographical bias 19
graphic representation in meta-analysis presentation 60
graphic results display in META program 77.
  See also analytical results display in META program
graphical presentation
  Cimetidine versus Placebo example 44, 45, 46
  Funnel plot 52
  Galbraith plot 47
  l'Abbè plot 50
  plot for sub-group analysis 53
  standard plots 44
graphics colors in META program 85
grey literature 9, 89

heterogeneity 89
  considerations on 39
  null hypothesis of 25
  quantifying 30, 42
  quantitative evaluation 30
  statistical 39
  See also test for heterogeneity

I^2 index 42
imprecision 24
inclusion criteria bias 18
independence of sources 21
indexing bias 18
Insert criteria button 74
Insert OR button 75
intention to treat analysis 12, 35, 90.
  See also per protocol analysis
interferon versus placebo (meta-analysis representation example) 61
internet-based search bias
  indexing bias 18
  search bias 18
inverse conformity publication bias 16
ITT. See intention-to-treat analysis

Klein formula
  for publication bias assessment 42
Klein's method 17

l'Abbè plot 50
  Cimetidine versus Placebo example 51
  See also Funnel plot; Galbraith plot

Index

legend setting in META program 86
log odds ratio estimation 48

Mantel-Haenszel method 26
   for confidence interval estimation 27
   pooled odds ratio estimation 28
   tests for heterogeneity 29
   variance estimation 28
   See also Peto method
maximum likelihood estimation 21
mean, weighted 24
medical bibliographic sources
   Embase 8
   Medline 8
medicine results using meta-analysis 1
Medline 8, 9
menu bar options
   Calculate 67
   Close 66
   Display/Analytic Results 67
   Display/Graphic Results 67
   Display/Variables 67
   Exit from Metanalysis 66
   File/New 66
   File/Open 66
   File/Save as... 66
   Options 67
   Select/Advanced select 66
   Select/All trials 66
   Select/Display/Execute SQL query 66
   Select/Simple select 66
meta-analysis
   abstracts inclusion and exclusion aspects 10
   application in biomedical field 4
   biases 15
   clinical research aspects 6
   cumulative 14, 45
   data accuracy aspects 34
   data collection for 11
   defined 90
   graphical representation 44
   heterogeneity considerations 39
   history 4
   involved statistical methods 13
   for medical data evaluation 2
   in medicine 1
   number needed to treat 43
   pooled effect evaluation 38
   published data collection 3
   randomized controlled trials and 59
   reading and evaluation 58
   representation examples 61
   results interpretation 14
   scoring systems 12
   statistical procedures used in 24
   as statistical test 3
   sub-group analysis 53
   synthesis of information 3
   test for publication bias 42
   trial output evaluation 35
   See also META program
meta-analysis planning 7
   clinical trials characteristics choosing 8
   outcomes planning 8
meta-analysis presentation 59
   graphic representation 60
   number needed to treat 60
   publication bias assessment 60
   sub-group analysis 60
   test for heterogeneity 60
meta-analyst caused bias
   extractor 19
   quality score 19
meta-analytic process aspects
   data reliability 9
   publication bias 9
META program
   characteristics 64
   installation 64
   risk factors description 69
   system requirements 64
   trial detail page 68
META program structure
   menu bar 65, 66
   status bar 67
   title bar 65
   tools bar 67
   See also menu bar options
META program, use of
   Advanced Select option 74
   all trials showing 76
   analytical results display 82
   file saving 72
   Fonts function 84
   graphics colors 85
   legend setting 86
   metanalysis file creation 70
   new trial addition 70
   Options function 84
   output on printer 80
   output on screen 77
   pre-existing trial modification 71
   showing of graphic results 77
   trials selection 72
metanalysis file
   creation 70
   saving 72

multiple publication bias 18
multiple used subjects bias 18

NNT. *See* number needed to treat
number needed to treat 14, 90
    Cimetidine versus Placebo example 43
    in meta-analysis presentation 60
    probabilistic approach 43
    quantitative approach 43
numeric output evaluation 35

odds ratio 13, 24, 26
    according to Gart 37
    according to Peto 37
    calculation 92
    defined 92
    for graphical presentation 44, 45
    in Funnel plot 52, 53
    Mantel-Haenszel method 27
    Peto method 29
    pooled 28, 45
    in publication bias 16
    for trials output evaluation 35, 37
    See also risk ratio
odds ratio calculation in fixed effects models
    Mantel-Haenszel method 26
    Peto method 29
odds ratio estimation in random effect
    models 30
Options function in META program 84
OR. *See* odds ratio
ORp. *See* pooled odds ratio
outcomes 12, 90
outcomes planning
    primary outcome 8
    secondary outcome 8
output evaluation, trial 35

PBA. *See* publication bias assessment
per protocol analysis 12, 35, 90. *See also*
    intention to treat analysis
percentage difference 26
Peto method
    for confidence interval estimation
      29
    tests for heterogeneity 29
    variance estimation 28
    See also Mantel-Haenszel method
Placebo. *See* Cimetidine versus Placebo
plot 90
    Funnel 52
    Galbraith 47
    l'Abbè 50

    for sub-group analysis 53
    standard 44
pooled effect 25, 26
pooled effect evaluation
    confidence interval estimation 39
    degrees of freedom 39
    natural logarithm of odds ratio 39
    odds ratio calculations 39
    standard error calculations 39
    test for heterogeneity 38, 39
pooled odds ratio 13
pooled odds ratio calculations
    for graphical presentation 45
    Mantel-Haenszel method 28
pooled risk difference 13, 43
PP analysis. *See* per protocol analysis
precision calculation
    Galbraith plot 48
    sub-group analysis 54
publication bias 9
    conformity 16
    inverse conformity 16
    quantitative evaluation 31
    test for 14
publication bias assessment
    Funnel plot for 43
    Klein formula 17, 42
    in meta-analysis presentation 60

Q test for homogeneity, Cochrane's 42
quality score 58
    bias 19
    defined 90
    information 12
quantifying heterogeneity
    I^2 index 42
    in random effects models 30
quantifying publication bias 31

random effects models 29, 89
    DerSimonian–Laird method application
      30
    difference of percentage 41
    log odds ratio estimation 41
    odds ratio calculation 30
    quantifying heterogeneity 30
    quantifying publication bias 31
    standard error estimation 41
    statistical heterogeneity and 40
    sub-group analysis 55
    See also fixed effects models
randomized controlled trials 9, 59
    defined 90

RCT. *See* randomized controlled trials
RD. *See* risk difference
RDp. *See* pooled risk difference
recording error bias 19
reference bias 18
reference databases 9
references search. *See* search for references technique
regression analysis 31
relative error 50
    Galbraith plot 48
relative risk estimation 26
REM. *See* random effects models
reporting bias 19
risk 90
risk difference 13
    calculation 91
    in publication bias 16
    See also pooled risk difference
risk difference estimation
    for graphical presentation 45
    for trials output evaluation 35, 36, 37
risk factors description
    Exposed–Events–Drop 69
    file format 69
risk ratio
    calculation 92
    in publication bias 16, 17
    See also odds ratio
RR. *See* risk ratio

sampling bias 16. *See also* selection bias; study bias
scientific paper reading
    abstract reading 10
    checklist for 10
    scoring system for 10
    title reading 10
scoring systems
    bias introduction 12
    quality score 12
    for scientific paper reading 10
    usage in meta-analysis 12
search bias 18
search for references technique
    capture–mark–recapture method 20
    Chapman method 21
    independence of sources 21
    maximum likelihood estimation 21
    sharks number estimation example 20
selected articles reading 11
selection bias 18. *See also* sampling bias; study bias

selector bias 18
sensitivity analysis 12, 13
sharks number estimation (example of references search) 20
Somatostatin example (sub-group analysis), 53
SQL, 74
standard error 26
    estimation 91
    in fixed effects models 26
    in Galbraith plot 47
statistical heterogeneity 39
    in fixed effect model 40
    in random effect model 40, 41
statistical methods
    odds ratio 13
    pooled odds ratio 13
    pooled risk difference 13
    risk difference 13
statistical procedures
    cumulative meta-analysis 14
    fixed effects models 13, 24
    number needed to treat 14
    random effects models 14, 29
    test for publication bias 14
statistical test for heterogeneity 13
study bias
    extractor 19
    quality score 19
    recording error 19
    reporting 19
    See also sampling bias; selection bias
sub-group analysis
    log odds ratio calculation 54
    in meta-analysis presentation 60
    plot for 53
    precision calculation 54
    Somatostatin example 53
synthesis of information 3
System Query Language 74
systematic research 92
systematic review 92

test for asymmetry of Funnel plot 53
test for heterogeneity 13, 25, 26, 39
    Cochrane's Q test 42
    Mantel-Haenszel method 29
    in meta-analysis presentation 60
    Peto method 29
    for pooled effect evaluation 38
test for publication bias 14
treatment of control group 12
treatment of study group 12

trial
   addition in META program, new 70
   comparison 12
   detail page 68
   information 12
   modification in META program, pre-existing 70
   output evaluation 35
   selection in META program 72
   showing in META program, all 76
trial detail page fields
   flags 68
   quality score 68
   symbol 68
   type of trial 68
trial results expressing as
   odds ratio (OR) 13
   risk difference (RD) 13

variance 24
variance estimation
   Mantel-Haenszel method 28
   Peto method 28

weight calculation 28
weighted mean 24